WHILE YOU QUIT

WHILE YOU QUIT

A SMOKER'S GUIDE TO REDUCING THE RISK OF HEART DISEASE AND STROKE

THEODORE FENSKE, MD
FOREWORD BY WILLIAM DAFOE, MD

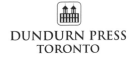

DUNDURN PRESS
TORONTO

Editor: Michael Carroll
Copy-editor: Ruth Chernia
Design: Courtney Horner
Printer: Webcom

Library and Archives Canada Cataloguing in Publication

Fenske, Theodore
    While you quit : a smoker's guide to reducing the risk
of heart disease and stroke / Theodore Fenske.

 Includes bibliographical references and index.
ISBN 978-1-55002-939-0

    1. Smoking cessation. 2. Cigarette smokers--Rehabilitation--
Handbooks, manuals, etc. 3. Cardiovascular system--Diseases.
I. Title.

RA645.T62F45 2009   616.86'506   C2008-908044-0

1   2   3   4   5   13   12   11   10   09

  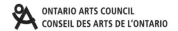

We acknowledge the support of the **Canada Council for the Arts** and the **Ontario Arts Council** for our publishing program. We also acknowledge the financial support of the **Government of Canada** through the **Book Publishing Industry Development Program** and **The Association for the Export of Canadian Books**, and the **Government of Ontario** through the **Ontario Book Publishers Tax Credit program**, and the **Ontario Media Development Corporation**.

Care has been taken to trace the ownership of copyright material used in this book. The author and the publisher welcome any information enabling them to rectify any references or credits in subsequent editions.

J. Kirk Howard, President

Published by Dundurn Press
Printed and bound in Canada
www.dundurn.com

Dundurn Press	Gazelle Book Services Limited	Dundurn Press
3 Church Street, Suite 500	White Cross Mills	2250 Military Road
Toronto, Ontario, Canada	High Town, Lancaster, England	Tonawanda, NY
M5E 1M2	LA1 4XS	U.S.A. 14150

For Oliver, Cameron, and Joel:
there is no greater joy a father could have.

CONTENTS

FOREWORD

Imagine that you are about to have a Thanksgiving Day dinner with your family, some relatives, and a few neighbours. One of the family members is Peter, a feisty fifty-five-year-old man who enjoys his food, his drink (albeit in moderation), and his cigarettes. Peter is sensitive to today's norms and excuses himself before and after the meal in order to smoke. The dinner is superbly cooked, and everyone has a most festive time. The dinner ends, the dishes are finally put away, the kids are playing outside, and everyone retires to the living room for further discussion. Politics, sports, and the latest scandals are all discussed. But, a number of family members are concerned that Peter is still smoking. You see, Peter's brother died prematurely of a heart attack, and everyone is worried about Peter, especially given his high risks for having a heart attack.

One of your other guests is Dr. Ted Fenske, a cardiologist, raconteur, and expert in the prevention of heart disease. Dr. Fenske "walks the talk" with his own superb lifestyle. In our fictional after-dinner discussion, Dr. Fenske is akin to a friendly, avuncular, family doctor who contributes his humour, wisdom, expertise, and gentle persuasion to the conversation.

The format of this book follows our patient Peter and Dr. Fenske as they both struggle with the complex issues facing the patient who is still addicted to smoking. Just as the patient is part of a social system (e.g., family, society), smoking is but one of the toxic ingredients that contribute to vascular disease. In addition to smoking, the traditional and newer risk factors are discussed. But this is not the usual litany of "what not to do." As Marcel Proust, the French novelist, said: "The real voyage of discovery consists not in seeking new lands, but in seeing with new eyes."

Part of these new "new lands" is a modern depiction of the atherosclerotic process utilizing a PLAC diagram (P=platelets, L=lining, A=active inflammation, C=cholesterol core) showing the complex interplay of the risk factors. Rather than a dry recitation of facts and statistics, Dr. Fenske weaves an interesting monologue with Peter, his medical challenges, and his perceptions. For example, he discusses the complex synergy of oral health, smoking, and heart disease. He uses historical vignettes throughout the text and provides the added contextual knowledge that piques our interest to appreciate the nuances of medical developments or pharmaceuticals. For example, did you know that the word *nicotine* came from J. Nicot, the French Ambassador to Portugal in the mid-1500s who introduced tobacco to France?

Patients often seek in-depth educational materials that provide more of a discussion. This book presents an intelligent discussion of the risk factors for heart disease with a major focus for the individual who continues to smoke. Rather than stigmatize the recalcitrant smoker and offer platitudes that "you must quit entirely," Dr. Fenske presents a respectful series of perspectives that the patient and treating physician need to consider. Rather than just lecture that "smoking is bad," the complex effects of the constituents of cigarette smoke are presented. Implicit in these discussions is the modern day recognition of the "readiness-for-change" model as promulgated by the psychologists Prochaska and DiClemente.[1]

Who would enjoy reading this book? Any interested and thoughtful individual who is concerned about his or her heart health would benefit. Although patients with documented disease may be more motivated, the discussions will benefit all. Having treated many patients in cardiac rehabilitation and secondary prevention clinics, I would recommend this book for all such patients. The reading and reflections offered by this book allow a patient and family to come to a learned perspective on the need for smoking cessation, as well as other aspects for heart health.

Reading Dr. Fenske's book *While You Quit* allows us to see vascular risk with "new eyes." As we complete our fictional after dinner discussion, we are left with the feeling that we have experienced a "voyage of discovery."

William Dafoe, MD
Regional Director of Capital Health Cardiac Rehabilitation
Alberta Cardiac Institute

ACKNOWLEDGEMENTS

I would like to thank my wife, Tanya, for being my trusty backboard off of whom I have bounced ideas over the years, and for her continual and consistent support and behind-the-scenes shaping and editing of the manuscript from its earliest form.

I am very thankful for the vision and encouragement of Johanna Bates, whose confidence in this project inspired its completion. Her passion is reminiscent of William Hutchinson Murray's compelling assertion that, "Whatever you can do, or dream you can, begin it. / Boldness has genius, power, and magic in it."

I am indebted to Matthew Manera, editor, for his careful attention to the details of the manuscript, his gentle grammatical tutoring — improving the structure and mechanics of my writing and smoothing out the awkward bits, and for his invaluable insights into content and tone.

I am grateful to Anne Bougie, literary agent with Johanna Bates Literary Consultants, for the helpful suggestions, timely enthusiasm, and limitless energy that she so graciously brought to this project.

I so appreciate my cardiology colleagues at the Royal Alexandra Hospital, Edmonton, for inspiring exemplary patient care, and for keeping the CCU machine running smoothly, even when my wheels fell off. In particular, I am very thankful for Dr. William Dafoe's thoughtful review of the manuscript and for his many helpful medical suggestions.

I remain grateful to my patients, those who have successfully quit smoking, those in the process, and even those who have vowed never to stop. They have provided me with endless insights into how health gains can be wrought, no matter what the context. Their plethora of questions, concerns, and frank discussions have challenged my limited thinking about disease prevention, and rendered my arguments for health all the stronger.

A special thanks to Olive and Toots, who have reminded me of the importance of seeing the person behind the rings of smoke. (You can do it, ladies!)

INTRODUCTION

I gazed out my office window like a mole squinting out from the opening of its burrow. It was late in the afternoon on one of those picture-perfect, blue-sky days that sang "come out and play!" But my heaps of paperwork were crowding me off my desk and showing no sign of retreat, as my secretary added another stack to the swell. "The woods are dark and deep but I have miles to walk before I sleep" ... that is, if I can stay awake. So I waded into the ponderous pile, hoping that with Edmonton's long summer days there might still be some brief rays of sunshine to enjoy when I finished. As I pushed through the referral letters, I came across one request that caught my attention. A general practitioner wanted me to perform a treadmill stress test on a middle-aged gentleman and render an opinion regarding his risk for vascular disease. He was a professional driver and needed medical clearance to maintain his Class 1 driver's licence. Although he had no symptoms to suggest a heart ailment at the present, his family doctor was worried about his risk for developing atherosclerosis and wanted me to lend a hand to head it off at the pass. Very routine so far. But the letter went on to say that the patient's younger brother had recently died of a heart attack, and (this is the part that piqued my interest) that, despite this tragic death in the family, he remained an ardent smoker. In the referral letter the doctor had underlined, "he is not willing to quit."

Often we heart specialists feel a sense of impending failure when asked to assess someone who smokes. Negative thoughts filled my mind. "If he's still smoking, what's the point in seeing him? I mean, smoking increases the risk of heart disease, so what do I have to offer? It takes time to go over the health hazards of smoking, and he's likely heard it a million times already. He's obviously not interested in quitting, and ... it's such a beautiful day outside."

Maclean's highlighted this frustration in their April 2006 lead article entitled "Overeaters, Smokers, and Drinkers: The Doctor Won't See You Now." The piece was designed to shock people into adopting healthy behaviour, and profiled an outspoken medic who unashamedly stated that "as a society we can no longer afford to spend money on those who don't take responsibility for their own health."[1]

But few of us are as narrow-minded as this. Such an approach doesn't offer any viable solution to the smoking addiction and merely puts people's backs up, widening the chasm between those who are at risk and the available risk-reduction strategies. Yes, we all need to take responsibility for our health, but the 1.3 billion smokers on the planet are at highest risk for developing heart disease and stroke and need intensified support rather than abandonment.

"Smoking be damned!" I thought. "How about offering him some insight into how he can lower his risks despite his addiction? Sure, I would have to acknowledge his smoking addiction and encourage him to consider quitting ... this is my 'bounden duty' as an MD. But the focus of my attention would be on the ways he could reduce his risk for developing vascular disease — while he considers quitting." With a scribble of my pen I took up the gauntlet and jotted a note for my secretary to arrange an appointment.

The glory days of smoking are past. Nearly half of all living adults who have ever smoked have now quit. There's no need for you to be left holding the bag while everyone else is breathing easily. But don't worry, I'm not going to go into the usual tirade — "It's not too late to quit smoking; you don't have to join the staggering statistics of smoking-related death, disease, and disability. Quit smoking now, while there's still time to save yourself, Ebenezer Scrooge!" I mean, you've heard the scare mantra before. This is not a "quit-smoking-or-else" book. Half of my patients smoke, and so do many of my friends. I've learned that badgering them to quit does little more than irritate and alienate. Besides, vascular disease is a complex business and is related to a wide range of insults to which we expose our bodies throughout any given day — Tim Hortons, McDonald's, and Wendy's, to name but a few culinary kinds. Every waking moment our blood vessels are defending themselves against the onslaught of injuries to which we knowingly or otherwise are exposed (the thousands of chemicals in a single cigarette certainly add to the monster mix, so quitting shouldn't be put off indefinitely). But as important as smoking is as a risk factor for developing heart artery disease and stroke, it isn't the only factor. Sure, smoking ranks as the number one modifiable risk factor. The anti-smoking campaign pamphlets are stating the truth, but there are numerous other factors that also accelerate heart disease.

When it comes to blood vessel injury, it's also critical to consider the role of psychological stress, sleep deprivation, inactivity, abdominal fat, high blood pressure, and elevated cholesterol. These all play an important part in damaging our blood vessels, rendering them more prone to disease. Likewise, as critical as smoking cessation is for improving heart health, there are numerous other no-nonsense endeavours that we can incorporate into our daily lives to enhance vascular function and help stave off disease.

In Canada, health promotion is greatly under-appreciated and generally misunderstood. Many Canadians seem open to trade in our hard-won health-care system for the far inferior American model. And most of us don't give our enjoyment of health much thought or concern, until something comes along to threaten it or, worse, steal it away by disease or accident. Those who do consider their health now and again, tend to think of it along the lines of an "all or nothing" state. As with other things in a consumer society, health is commonly viewed like any other commodity, something we can possess. But our health is far from a possession that we can acquire and then forget about, shoving it onto some shelf to collect dust. What I hope to clarify in the following pages is a fuller and more realistic view of health: one that will both foster a better appreciation of health's fragility and encourage responsible stewardship.

Chapter 1 opens the discussion by outlining how we measure cardiovascular risk. This is square one for appreciating the risk-reduction approach to health. This discussion is a reference point for the chapters that follow, detailing the steps to reduce this risk in an incremental fashion. Rather than simply covering a behavioural "to do" list, or providing a litany of "not to dos," my hope is to outline the different ways our cardiovascular system is susceptible to disease and how its healthy function can be optimized. In my clinic, I will often sketch out a cartoon of a blood vessel wall to aid in my explanations (see the drawing of a cross-section of a blood vessel). Using such a simplified model, I highlight the four main layers or compartments where health and disease battle it out. This gives my patients a better handle on the wonders of vascular medicine and how they can be involved for health's sake. Using this visual model,

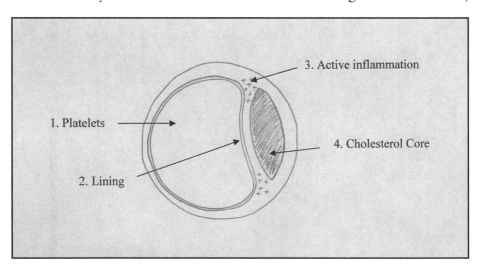

Figure 0.1: Blood vessel in cross-section.

I will focus attention on each compartment in turn and consider the dynamic balance of factors, both good and bad, that help determine our state of vascular health.

When it comes to preventing vascular injury, we don't have the luxury of unlimited time. To make hay while the sun shines, I begin discussions about the more time-sensitive areas of the vessel wall that need attention. Some health behaviours can pay dividends within days; others within weeks. Some can take months or even a year. We'll begin by covering the things that will deliver the most amount of benefit in the least amount of time. This way you can expect to reduce your risks ASAP.

Our health is more of a journey than a destination point. As such, vascular health can best be enhanced by taking a series of intentional steps in the same direction, rather than expecting it to arrive as a package. The key is to understand the priorities of heart health and to get started. The ambition of this book is to show you the variety of on-ramps you can take to the road of improved vascular health, even if quitting isn't on the map at present.

1

RISKY BUSINESS

Risk Perceptions

Most parents with teenagers will agree that youth have a skewed concept of risk-taking. It's all about now, tonight, this girl, that dare. It's an all-or-nothing world, and consequences are as far away as the moon. When it comes to cruising down main street on Friday night, Bob Seger pretty much summed things up with "we've got tonight … who needs tomorrow." So there's a good reason teens have higher car insurance premiums and there is merit for raising the driving age further. But adults also can have misperceptions about risk. We tend to get hot and bothered about remote possibilities off in the distance, and neglect the real monsters staring us in the face. To better appreciate the real perils in this threatening world, we need to take a look at the big picture. When we call in the statisticians to do the actual body count, it isn't the West Nile Virus, mad cow disease, or the Avian flu that's doing us in; more Canadians died of heart disease and stroke this past year than all other causes combined.[1]

And the forecast for this coming year looks no better.

One in four Canadians suffers from heart disease. With over 75,000 heart attacks and 25,000 strokes each year, the number-one killer we have to worry about is vascular disease, not lightning strikes or sharks. Although advances in high-tech treatments continue to improve the survival rate of those people who suffer from heart attacks, the overall death rate still exceeds 50 percent, underscoring the need for preventative strategies. It is wise to limit exposure to morose mosquitoes, crazy cows, and foul fowl, of course, but, more importantly, we need to reduce the number of hits we take to our vulnerable cardiovascular system.

The Consultation

I was running behind in a full clinic when I finally saw Mr. Peter H., the devoted smoker whose brother had just died of a heart attack. Peter was a long-haul truck driver in his mid-fifties, heavy set, with labourer's hands and a five o'clock shadow, even though it wasn't yet noon. He was accompanied by his eldest daughter, who was studying nursing at our local college. She was keen to learn about her father's health status and wanted to be as involved as she could. Despite her encouragement, however, Peter appeared uncomfortable about being "the patient." With arms folded across his large chest and eyes shielded by the rim of his baseball cap, he leaned against the examination table, reminding me of a bouncer from my adolescent pub-crawling days. I introduced myself with an enthusiastic handshake and commented on the weather, because that's what we talk about on the prairies. A grunt is all I got out of him. He shifted his weight to the other foot as if to say "I hate being here, so quit the small talk and get on with it." Since we were off to a bit of a stuttering start, I tried one of my favourite doctor-patient bonding manoeuvres.

"I'm a Class 1 driver, too, you know," I offered eagerly, holding out my licence to prove my credentials.

"Whatever," he mumbled as he continued to stare down at the floor uncomfortably, then blurted out, "My brother saw a heart specialist, too. He got a bunch of tests done, but it didn't stop him from dying of a heart attack two months later."

One of the most disturbing parts of vascular disease is its unpredictability. As important as the developments of high-tech diagnostics and state-of-the-art treatments have been for management of people suffering from heart attacks and stroke, you still have to be mostly alive to benefit. The latest clot-buster therapies and angioplasty balloons have substantially reduced the risk of dying of a heart attack, but are like "all the king's horses and all the king's men" if you're DOA. Nothing we have developed to date has been able to reduce the sudden death rate related to vascular disease. This is why we need to work on preventing these catastrophes. Only in this way will we be able to meaningfully address the enormous burden heart disease and stroke place on our society.

"Half of people with heart attacks die suddenly, before they even reach medical care," I related to Peter and his daughter. "Don't forget our late, great John Candy. He had a bad family history of early heart disease and, although he had quit smoking, he died without any warning of a massive heart attack during a movie shoot in Mexico. Despite his international stardom, nothing could be done for him. That's part of the reason your doc wanted me to see you — to decrease your risk of having a fate similar to your brother's."

The Shock and Awe of Vascular Accidents

I know all too well the sudden and unexpected nature of vascular disease. I've seen it enough in the emergency department: family and friends huddled together and grieving, gathered around their loved one, who only minutes earlier was talking, laughing, and full of life like the rest of us, now dead. But I've felt the sting of this disease process as well. In August 2004, I experienced what it feels like to be struck down by vascular disease — and as a wannabe poster boy for health, it was the shock of my life.

While I was at the height of my cardiology career, and basking in excellent health and good fortune, I suffered a massive stroke. There were no warning signs or symptoms; disaster descended out of the blue sky. I was only forty at the time and I figured that because I didn't smoke, was in excellent physical condition, followed a vegetarian diet, and didn't have high blood pressure, high cholesterol, or high blood sugars, my risk of vascular disease was rock-bottom low. In fact, I had just qualified for the Boston Marathon with my personal best time and I felt like Superman. Then boom! While playing tag with my three boys at our neighbourhood park, I was suddenly face down in the sand, bewildered. Why was I having so much difficulty getting up? It confused me that I couldn't use my arm. When I tried to stand I overheard my eldest son yelling to my wife for help, "There's something wrong with Daddy! He isn't moving right, and he's scaring me with his face!" My wife instantly noticed my facial droop and the difficulty I was having walking, dragging my left leg like some kind of pirate. Her words stunned me, "I'm calling the ambulance. I think you're having a stroke!"

The declaration pained my ears like some kind of dissonant chord. "Having a what?" Me, having a stroke? It was like some bad dream where crazy things happen that make no sense, and you're powerless to change them. "I don't think so" I argued. "My arm doesn't move because … well … because I must have bumped my funny bone, that's all. It'll be fine. There's no need to bother with an ambulance … besides it will frighten the boys … it's nothing … really."

Fortunately, my wife didn't buy that John Wayne "it's really nothing" line. The ambulance arrived at the scene within minutes and sped me to the hospital where the emergency team made the diagnosis. As it turned out, the main blood vessel in my neck, called the carotid artery, had somehow torn. The innermost lining of the artery had ripped away from the rest of the wall where it normally lies anchored. This kind of tear or *dissection*, as we doctors call it, is a real disaster. Damage to this inner lining exposes the other, deeper layers of the blood vessel wall to the circulating blood. Within seconds, blood clots form on the injured section. Now, if you cut yourself shaving, that's just fine. You want blood to clot to stop the bleeding from your chin, so you don't have to have bits of tissue stuck to your face all day. But blood clotting inside the carotid artery? Nothing less than a disaster. In my case, so much blood clot formed in my neck artery that it plugged it completely and stopped the flow of blood to part of my brain. Over 80 percent of those unfortunate enough to suffer this type of stroke don't live to tell the tale. If I hadn't received lifesaving therapy in record time, I would have surely added to these grim statistics.

Why Bad Things, Like Heart Attacks and Strokes, Happen to Good People

My stroke was a freak accident. It was like being struck by lightning on a sunny day or getting snow in Alabama. Although this type of stroke (the spontaneous tearing of a blood vessel), is more common in young people, it is generally a rare and unusual event. The odds of this happening to you are 200,000 to 1 — similar to winning any prize in a Canadian lottery. So it's not something you have to spend any time worrying about. To date, I've received no good explanation as to why this stroke happened to me, and I may never get an answer. As I stated, I was as healthy as could be. My only dietary sins involved the killing of fresh carrots, fruit plate gluttony, and the occasional coveting of someone else's salad choice. My habits included daily exercise and Tai Chi, and my only addiction was the runner's high. And since I've never understood what it was that precipitated my stroke, I've never been sure how to avoid a replay. This "not knowing" has created a certain level of mistrust in my body and a foreboding about my future. Fortunately, this is not the case for most vascular diseases. We *do* know what causes the vast majority of blood vessel injuries and how to reduce them. So you don't have to have a cloud hanging over your head wondering if and when a heart attack or stroke is coming your way. There is action that can be taken.

Our understanding of heart health has changed substantially over the years. In the past, heart conditions were often misdiagnosed as gastrointestinal ailments or ascribed to the nineteenth-century catch-all term, "consumption." Even with the dawn of the scientific age, heart disease remained shrouded in mystery. It wasn't until 1912 that crushing chest pain was recognized as a heart attack symptom, and many thought that heart problems were caused by physical exertion. Clarence DeMar, the seven-time winner of the Boston Marathon was advised not to compete because of concerns he might precipitate a heart condition. "I was told I had a heart murmur and shouldn't run, and that I'd feel weak going up and down stairs," he said to reporters after completing his thirty-second marathon in 1928. He went on to say, "I've been looking for these symptoms for over a quarter of a century now and I've been feeling fine. But recently I heard that the old doctor, who told me I shouldn't run, died of heart failure himself. So I've often wondered if he wasn't listening to his own heart by mistake."[2] With little else to offer, bed rest for upwards of two to three months was the mainstay of therapy for all patients with suspected heart disease, and they either recovered patiently or died of boredom.

It wasn't until those happy days of the 1960s that our lifestyle choices were recognized as playing a role in causing heart disease. While the media was reporting on the Bay of Pigs fiasco, and many of us were "splish splashing" on our Saturday nights, Dr. Thomas Royle Dawber coined the term *risk factors* when he brought attention to what are currently accepted as conventional determinants of heart disease. In his landmark study of disease patterns in a New England population, he recognized for the first time that smoking, as well as high blood pressure, elevated cholesterol levels, diabetes, inactivity, and psychological stress, increases the likelihood of heart disease.[3] And this finding is by no means confined to the eastern seaboard of the United States. These same risk factors have the made-in-

Canada stamp on them as well. In fact, no matter where on the planet you may want to hide, these same risk factors will find you. A Canadian-based investigation team has recently illustrated the strong relationship between Dr. Dawber's conventional risk factors and the incidence of heart disease in fifty-two countries.[4] According to their data, nearly 90 percent of all heart attacks can be explained by nine key risk factors.

Global Risk Factors

- smoking
- high blood pressure
- diabetes
- abdominal obesity
- psychological stress
- low dietary fibre
- inactivity
- alcohol in extreme
- high cholesterol

Source: "The Interheart Study." *Lancet* 364 (2004): 937–52.

Newer risk contenders are continually vying for position on this list with the promise of better predicting who is at greater risk for developing heart disease. But, to date, they have been disappointing, and have offered little beyond the nine listed. Woody Allen's movie *Sleeper* parodied the evolution of medical dogma, portraying life two hundred years in the future, with doctors recommending smoking, fatty foods, and sedentary living as heart-healthy choices. But in the real world of cardiovascular risk factors, the more things change, the more they stay the same. The mechanism of vascular disease may be complex, but the relationship between risk factors and heart disease is ironclad in the scientific literature and only getting further support as we learn more about this disease.

Predicting Risk

In the words of Yogi Berra, "predictions are difficult, especially about the future." While no one can reliably predict your risk of having a heart attack or stroke today or tomorrow, there are methods of reasonably estimating the risk of one of these events over the coming decade. Medics want to know this risk estimate so they can direct their attention to those people at greatest risk. And you can use a risk estimate to gauge your progress as you make inroads on your health path.

The more risk factors you have, the greater the chance that a heart attack or stroke will come a-knockin'. But not all risk factors are created equal, for all people. For example, smoking increases the risk for vascular disease more in a young person than in the aged. So rather than simply adding risk factors, we make use of statistical weighting in the risk calculation to improve the predictive value. The most popular risk calculator, and the one I use with my patients daily, is the Framingham Risk Score.[5] It remains the gold standard for estimating risk in populations such as we have in Canada, and is fast and straightforward to use. All you need to do is plug in the numbers from five easily measured risk parameters. The first two are your age and your smoking status. These, of course, you can fill in right now. The remaining three require a blood pressure check and a blood test to measure your cholesterol level. Points are accumulated depending upon your measurements. The higher the point score, the higher the risk of having a heart attack within the next decade. The tallied point score correlates with a ten year percentage risk. Estimates less than 10 percent are considered low; 10 to 20 percent, intermediate; and above 20 percent, high risk for having a heart attack.

When we look at the parameters of the Framingham risk score on page 29, we see that age racks up the most points. It makes sense that the older you are, the higher your risk. It should be emphasized, however, that, although the likelihood of vascular disease increases with age, heart disease is not limited to the elderly. Half of heart attacks and one-third of strokes occur in those under sixty-five years of age. Even children have evidence of blood vessel disease. A forerunner of vascular plaque is thought to be the "fatty streak," a deposit of lipid in the vessel wall that can come and go over time. Autopsy studies from motor-vehicle-accident fatalities have even shown fatty streaks in the heart arteries of children, indicating that vascular disease is everyone's business. But because atherosclerosis is typically the result of repeat offense to the vessels, the older you are, the greater the disease burden. But it's never too late to reduce risk.

Men

Estimation of 10-year risk of nonfatal myocardial infarction or coronary death (Framingham Heart Study) in men

Age in years	Points
20–34	-9
35–39	-4
40–44	0
45–49	3
50–54	6
55–59	8
60–64	10
65–69	11
70–74	12
75–79	13

Cholesterol level (mmol/L)	Age in years (points)				
	20–39	40–49	50–59	60–69	70–79
≤4.14	0	0	0	0	0
4.15–5.19	4	3	2	1	0
5.2–6.19	7	5	3	1	0
6.2–7.2	9	6	4	2	1
>7.21	11	8	5	3	1

Smoking Status	Age in years (points)				
	20–39	40–49	50–59	60–69	70–79
Nonsmoker	0	0	0	0	0
Smoker	8	5	3	1	1

High-density lipoprotein cholesterol level (mmol/L)	Points
≥1.55	-1
1.30–1.54	0
1.04–1.29	1
<1.04	2

Systolic blood pressure (mmHg)	Untreated (points)	Treated (points)
<120	0	0
120–129	0	1
130–139	1	2
140–159	1	2
≥160	2	3

Points total	10-year risk (%)
1	1
2	1
3	1
4	1
5	2
6	2
7	3
8	4
9	5
10	6
11	8
12	10
13	12
14	16
15	20
16	25
17	>30

Estimation of 10-year risk can also be made at hin.nhlbi.nih. gov/atpiii/calculator.asp

Women

Estimation of 10-year risk of nonfatal myocardial infarction or coronary death (Framingham Heart Study) in women

Age in years	Points
20–34	-7
35–39	-3
40–44	0
45–49	3
50–54	6
55–59	8
60–64	10
65–69	12
70–74	14
75–79	16

Cholesterol level (mmol/L)	Age in years (points)				
	20–39	40–49	50–59	60–69	70–79
≤4.14	0	0	0	0	0
4.15–5.19	4	3	2	1	1
5.2–6.19	8	6	4	2	1
6.2–7.2	11	8	5	3	2
>7.21	13	10	7	4	2

Smoking status	Age in years (points)				
	20–39	40–49	50–59	60–69	70–79
Nonsmoker	0	0	0	0	0
Smoker	9	7	4	2	1

High-density lipoprotein cholesterol level (mmol/L)	Points
≥1.55	-1
1.30–1.54	0
1.04–1.29	1
<1.04	2

Systolic blood pressure (mmHg)	Untreated (points)	Treated (points)
<120	0	0
120–129	1	3
130–139	2	4
140–159	3	5
≥160	4	6

Points total	10-year risk (%)
<9	1
9	1
10	1
11	1
12	1
13	2
14	2
15	3
16	4
17	5
18	6
19	8
20	11
21	14
22	17
23	22
24	27
≥25	>30

Estimation of 10-year risk can also be made at hin.nhlbi.nih. gov/atpiii/calculator.asp

As you might have guessed, smoking contributes to the point score in a big way. In fact, the point score you get with smoking is similar to the points from aging ten years. It's not only the facial complexion that prematurely ages when we smoke, it's also the unseen, all-important blood vessels that age, as well. The good news about smoking and vascular disease is that the risk drops dramatically once you quit. So the risk number you tally today isn't carved in stone. As part of my motivational address, I often use the risk-assessment tool to illustrate the positive impact quitting can have on the risk number. Smoking is such a big risk factor that it can bump a low-risk score up into an intermediate one, or an intermediate score into a high-risk one. Check out Peter's results:

Peter's Risk Score

Risk Parameter	Points with smoking	Points without smoking
Age	6	6
Smoking status	3	0
Blood pressure	1	1
Total cholesterol	2	2
HDL cholesterol	2	2
Total points	14	11
10-year risk range	10–20%	< 10%

But it's not all bad news. In fact there is a great deal of good news about butting out ASAP. Within eight hours of quitting there is a measurable improvement in oxygen delivery to our tissues. You can't even fly to Europe in eight hours (at my airport you often don't even take off in that period of time), but your body has started repairing from a lifetime of insult on the lungs. This means that after an eight-hour sleep, you've already made some headway on health. Keep that in mind before you give in to the first-thing-in-the-morning cigarette. Not impressed yet? Take a look at the figure on the benefits over time of quitting and scan to the 24-hour point on the time axis. Here the risk of dying from a heart attack is already less than it was at baseline. Nothing I know can reduce vascular risk so quickly or dramatically as quitting smoking.[7] By this time tomorrow, a smoke-free day will pay measurable risk benefit dividends (allow an extra half hour in Newfoundland).

Our lungs begin to recuperate by the two-week mark. This is why surgeons are so keen about patients holding off on cigarettes for two weeks before going under the knife, since this is the most effective way to reduce the risk of getting lung infection at and around the time of surgery. Without the insult of cigarette smoke, mucous production goes back to normal and the lungs' ability to remove inhaled particles, including bacteria, improves remarkably. By three months, the extra risk that smoking adds to developing heart disease has plummeted to 50 percent. It's like a Boxing Day sale! You don't say "no" to half-price power tools, mixers, or stereo equipment. Why say "no" to your health? But wait, it gets even better. At two years of smoke-free life, your risk of vascular disease is very similar to that of your non-smoking neighbour, and even your non-smoking twin. Without an upper age limit for these benefits to be reaped, it's never too late to quit![6]

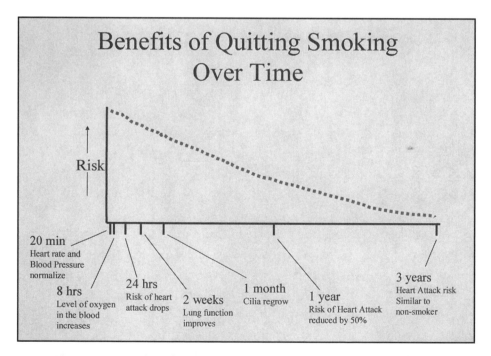

Figure 1.1: Benefits of quitting smoking over time. Courtesy of T.K. Fenske, "Preventing the Next Heart Attack." *Patient Care* 15(8) (August 2004): 44–53.

Genetic Influences

The reason why some get heart disease can't be fully explained by adding up risk factors. First, not everyone has vascular risk factors. (Mind you, it's getting harder to find such risk-free people since 80 percent of Canadians have at least one major risk factor.) Nonetheless, some people wind up with heart disease despite absent risk factors. They follow careful diets and do all the right things, but succumb at an early age despite the best of intentions (take me, for instance). Second, not everyone who is at risk for heart disease ends up getting a heart attack. There are those who enjoy long and productive lives despite having significant vascular risk factors. The late George Burns is a prime example, cracking one hundred years with stogie in hand, proving that nature can sometimes triumph over nurture. So to explain why some do or don't get the bad disease, we need to consider the genetic predisposition to vascular disease. If the genetic substrate sets the stage, then bad actors, like hypertension, smoking, or high cholesterol, can run amuck and ruin the show.

Heart disease and stroke tend to run in families. This is especially true for identical twins. When both babies originate from the same fertilized egg, they share exact copies of DNA. Identical twins not only look the same on the outside, but they are also built from the same blueprint. It's not surprising, then, that they might share similarities in both health and disease. Studies have shown that if one identical twin develops vascular disease, the risk of a heart attack is extraordinarily high in the other: eight times higher for the identical brother and fifteen times higher for the identical sister. The more genetically similar we are, the more likely we will be susceptible to the same disease processes, heart disease included. But it's not just a problem for twins. The Framingham Offspring study of 1971, involving over 2,300 subjects, helped define this genetic influence on family members in general.[8] They found that heart disease in first-degree relatives (which includes mom, dad, brother, or sister) doubles the other family members' risk of developing vascular disease. This is especially true if they were younger when they developed their disease: younger than fifty-five years of age for men and sixty-five for women. We refer to this as having a positive family history. Contrary to the common usage of the word "positive" in reference to our self-actualizing, you-can-do-it culture, "positive" in medical circles is always a bad thing. The fact that my patient, Peter, had a younger brother with heart disease is sobering and ends up doubling his risk of something similar as recalculated below. If you've got a positive family history, beware! As Spanish philosopher, George Santayana said, "Those who cannot learn from history are doomed to repeat it."

Peter's Updated Risk Score

Framingham Risk Score (%)	x	Family History (1 if negative or 2 if positive)	=	10-Year Cardiovascular Risk

Peter:

10–20%	x	2	=	> 20% (High Risk)

But it's not all a matter of fate. The role of our genetic makeup in our health is far from hard and fast and is, in fact, quite dynamic. How we treat our bodies, and what we expose ourselves to day to day, can play a significant role in how our genes are employed. In 1953, Watson and Crick discovered the double helix spiral-staircase structure of DNA, laying the foundation for genetic investigations of life's blueprint. Now fifty years later, the Human Genome Project has decoded this molecule of life, ordering no less than three billion building-block chemicals to define its structure. And out of these efforts has come a growing understanding that our genes are sensitive to environmental cues. So it's not just the genetic code that's remarkable; it's how the code gets read as we interact with our surroundings. Just like the success of a joke depends upon how the words are spoken, our vascular health depends upon more than just the molecular sequence of our genetic code, but how the code is used by our bodies.

The study of how our genes are managed by our cells is referred to as epigenetics. This field of research investigates the *how* and *why* of gene expression: how genes are unravelled and why certain sequences are *read* while others are packaged up and stored away. The role of epigenetics is to genes as Brian Epstein was to the Beatles. Affectionately considered the "fifth Beatle," Epstein's tireless efforts to secure recording contracts and promote the quartet at ever-larger venues were largely responsible for the group's early success. Management of any enterprise is critical to its optimal functioning, genetic activity included. Recent studies have revealed that there are certain physical conditions that *turn on* the expression of some genes, and *turn off* the expression of others. This selection of which genes are read and which ones are shelved can have profound effects on our blood vessel health, since some genes are protective, while others can be harmful. The state of high blood pressure, for example, can influence our DNA management system and silence production of protective proteins, which can result in vascular injury. The flipside is also true: regular exercise, for example, turns on protective gene sequences that can help in vascular repair. It's pretty heady stuff. Our gene storage logistics are enough to make IKEA furniture designers cringe, and our cellular DNA strand compression system outshines anything that even Bill Gates could imagine. Fortunately, we don't have to understand the intricacies to reap the benefits. But it's worthwhile knowing this: things we do or fail to do can have an important impact on our health by modifying how our genes are expressed. So if your family history is dismal, take heart. Depending upon your day-to-day choices, you can carve out a much healthier path than your forebears did.

What's Hot and What's Not

Knowing a little family history and tallying up risk factors can help us predict the threat of heart disease, but they fail to explain what triggers the problem. Why did the heart attack or stroke happen today, instead of yesterday, or last week? The precipitating factors of vascular events are not completely understood. In the movies, heart attacks are often set off by sexual intercourse, as in *Private Benjamin* or by intense emotional stress, as portrayed by Richard Dreyfuss in *Once Around*. It makes for better entertainment, but doesn't explain the 99 percent of incidents that occur without such melodramatics, seemingly out of the blue. Although we do see an increase in heart attacks during the cold months (in Edmonton, Alberta, that's early September through late May), and after a heavy snow fall (when sedentary NHL fans try to quickly clear the driveway during commercial breaks), understanding the precise trigger has remained out of reach.

When we examine a blood vessel up close and search out the plaques that stud its diseased surface, we see that they differ in size, shape, and content. Some of these plaques are more prone to breaking and allowing blood to clot on their surfaces than others. One of the reasons is that some plaques are busier with metabolic activity than others. The more the metabolic flurry in the wall of the artery, the more likely "it's gonna blow, Captain." This susceptibility to break or rupture is referred to as *plaque vulnerability*, and helps to explain what precipitates a heart attack or stroke. Because of the increased goings-on in the wall of the blood vessel, vulnerable plaques have higher temperatures than their neighbouring, more calm and collected, stable plaques. Using micro-thermometers placed inside the arteries of the heart, it is possible to actually measure this increased temperature. The hotter plaques are more likely to break, rupture, and cause calamity, while the cooler ones remain "steady as she goes." But who wants a temperature probe stuck into their heart arteries to find out their cardiovascular risk? Not a particularly practical screening tool to offer the public.

Other technologies have been advanced to help identify vulnerable plaques. Computed tomography, or CT scanning, has been touted as a viable means to identify high-risk patients. I've had many patients who have had CT calcium scoring done by a private lab in the United States, asking me to interpret the results for them and determine their risk level. Unfortunately, CT imaging only tells us whether or not calcified plaques are present on our heart arteries. It doesn't tell us if those plaques are hotties or just cold fish. It's less important to know about the *presence* of vascular plaque, than it is to know about the *stability* of that plaque. Most of us have some degree of plaque formation just quietly sitting there in our arterial walls. Even our children have fatty streaks lining their blood vessels. While it is good to have no plaque in our vasculature, not all plaques will go on to produce symptomatic disease. More valuable than simply demonstrating the presence of arterial plaque, is determining the metabolic activity of that plaque.

During my medical school training, I spent a summer studying a brand new technology called Positron Emission Tomography (it took me a while to say that mouthful, too). My "PET project," as I called it, was to investigate various applications of this high-tech imaging device, and it kept me mostly out of trouble. Using radioactive tracers, PET imaging can measure metabolic activity in our bodies, without the need for invasive temperature probes. It's still a long way from Dr. McCoy's diagnostic tricorder in *Star Trek*, but nonetheless, when we image blood vessels with this super camera, the metabolically active plaques on our blood vessels light up. It's been shown that people at highest risk for heart disease have more of these hot spots on their arteries, like time bombs ready to go off. But this expensive and cumbersome technology is a research tool only, and not something that can be easily incorporated into routine medical practice.

There has been considerable interest in providing a simple and cost-effective means to identify these vulnerable plaques in clinical medicine. Fortunately, this can be done, albeit indirectly. And we don't need to place thermometers in our heart arteries or undergo radioactive imaging studies. All we need to do is get hold of a measuring tape and bare our bellies.[9] (See Figure 1.2.) The explanation is detailed in Chapter 6 and describes the central role of our belly fat when it comes to raising the temperatures of our vulnerable vascular plaques. Suffice it to say here, our risk of heart attack and stroke rises substantially if we're losing the battle of the bulge. Waist circumference thresholds for this problem have been estimated to be 102 cm (40 inches) for men and 88 cm (35 inches) for women. If your midriff measures more than this, your risk of vascular disease is doubled. Certain ethnic groups, including South and East Asians, are even more sensitive to excess abdominal fat, and therefore the thresholds for concern are lower for them: 90 cm (36 inches) for men and 80 cm (32 inches) for women.[10]

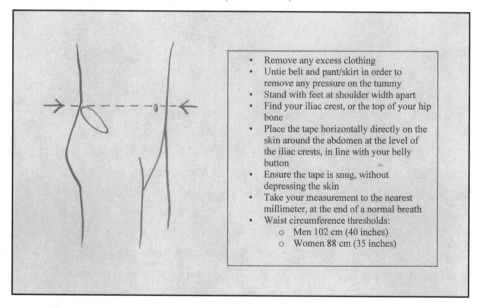

Figure 1.2: Measuring waist circumference.

More Than a Number

The following equation can be used to put a number on your risk. To estimate your risk of heart attack or stroke over the next ten years, first plug in your values on the Framingham Risk Score

(FRS). Then figure if your family history is positive (you have a mother or sister who developed vascular disease under the age of sixty-five years, or a father or brother who developed the disease under the age of fifty-five years), and if so, multiply the FRS by two. Lastly, measure your waist circumference. If your tummy exceeds the thresholds listed, then to arrive at the final estimate you need to multiply the FRS by a factor of two, once more. The complete risk assessment equation looks something like this: Framingham Risk Score (%) x Family History (1 if negative or 2 if positive) x Waist Circumference (1 if under threshold or 2 if over threshold) = 10-year cardiovascular risk.

The point of estimating vascular risk is not to instill fear or guilt, but to serve as a reality check about the fragility of our health and a reference point for health improvement actions. The risk estimate that we arrive at by using the above equation isn't fixed. We can reduce risk if we know what specific steps need taking, and take them. Otherwise what's the point? As Ebenezer Scrooge in Dickens's *A Christmas Carol* asked of the third spectre, "Answer me one question. Are these the shadows of the things that *Will be*. Or are they shadows of the things that *May be*. Men's courses will foreshadow certain ends.... But if the courses be departed from, the ends will change. Why show me this, if I am past all hope?"

Yes, there is considerable hope. With some attention, the risk of developing heart disease or stroke can be significantly reduced. The hope of this book is to provide a rationale for health interventions that can offset some of the negative effects of smoking on the vasculature, even while the cigarette defiantly smolders between your lips. Chapters that follow will outline the four specific illness-causing mechanisms that are known to accelerate vascular disease and detail the practical changes that you can make in your daily routine to foster health, while you quit.

2

BLOOD IS THICKER THAN WATER

Doin' It Right on the Wrong Side of Town

My flight to New Orleans was delayed by bad weather, extending my travel time from eight hours to over fourteen. When I finally got to the hotel I was itching to get outside for some fresh air. I knew that I didn't have much time before nightfall, but the late afternoon sun was still warm, and I really needed to stretch my legs. The French Quarter was my destination of choice. I figured that running the perimeter of that square-mile tourist landmark would be an ideal way to loosen up before dinner. But the best-laid plans of mice and men often go awry — I got myself lost. Some construction forced me to alter my route, and then the sun went down — not the dependable, dawdling sundown as in the true north strong and free — it just disappeared! One minute it was daylight; the next I was staring down dark streets and abandoned alleys that all looked frustratingly similar, one to the next, but desperately unfamiliar at the same time. And I'm not the only one staring. "Hey chicken legs!" I hear from across the street. "You think you're superman?" I quickly stopped to ask an elderly black lady for directions. "Oh my dear!" she exclaimed, "*You* shouldn't be out here at night." But before she could direct me, I heard over my shoulder, "Run, Forrest, Run!" So I did, and I didn't stop running until somehow I was back in my hotel room.

Generally, going for a jog is a considered healthy activity, which I passionately endorse. Habitual exercise has been shown to reduce the risks of vascular disease and improve longevity. But *that* particular run on the wrong side of the tracks wasn't doing my long-term survival any good. "Downright foolish," my wife exclaimed when I returned, pale-faced and trembling. "Next time," she insisted, "use the hotel gym. That way you can still exercise, but you won't have to worry about getting lost in the dark somewhere unsafe."

My running experience in Nawlins reminded me of "bad" blood clots. We need to be able to form blood clots. Without them, shaving in the morning or peeling carrots for lunch would be highly hazardous activities. But heart attacks and strokes occur because blood clots form in the wrong place at the wrong time. Timing and location can make the difference between appropriate control of blood loss when we cut ourselves using a potato peeler and a life-threatening heart attack when the clot forms on one of our heart arteries. To reduce the risk of a vascular catastrophe we need to reduce the body's blood-clotting response. But it's a fine line. We don't want to prevent blood clots from forming completely, we just want to reduce them. To reduce our risk of heart attack or stroke we need to achieve that hallowed middle ground — blood "thin" enough to avoid clotting off our heart arteries yet "thick" enough to keep us from bleeding to death from life's bumps and bruises. The trick is to prevent the bad blood clots (the ones that lead to heart attack or stroke), while not messing too much with the good ones (the potato-peeler cuts and shaving nicks).

Red, White, and Glue

The first time I took a close look at blood I was eleven years old. My dad had an old monocular microscope — the kind with a mirror at the base that reflects light onto the viewing platform. It was memorable because it was my first time using a microscope and because my brother got the blood sample from pricking *my* finger with the needle. As we peered down through the lens at the red smudge, an entire microscopic universe came into focus. Under low power magnification, the various blood cells caught the reflected light and reminded me of looking through a kaleidoscope with myriad patterns and colours. Under higher magnification we were able to make out individual cells, a skill I would later hone in medical school. The red blood cells dominated the view, like old-fashioned red bingo chips scattered on the table. Up close, we could see their smooth, round shape that gives them the ability to slip and slide through the miles of blood vessels in our bodies and squeeze into the smallest capillaries to deliver oxygen to our tissues.

But that wasn't all we saw. Every once in a while, as we scanned the microscopic playing field of red cells, we would spot a transparent glob. These larger cells were harder to see than the red cells, and were larger in size, with irregular shapes. I later learned that what we were seeing were white blood cells — the cells that carry out surveillance functions in our bodies and guard against infection. For us novice observers, the red and white blood cells were all we appreciated. But with a trained eye and some enhancing staining techniques, a third type of microscopic body is visible: the platelet (pronounced "plate-let"). It is these cell fragments that are responsible for blood clotting. If we could have examined my pricked finger up close, we would have been able to see them at work, all bunched together at the site of the needle injury to stop the bleeding.

Platelets are the first responders at the scene of vascular injury. Like the Dutch boy with his finger in the dike, the primary job of the platelet is to plug holes in our blood vessel walls. These cell fragments were discovered in the mid-1800s when biologists noticed peculiar little clumps that formed at the site of blood vessel incisions. About a fifth the size of a red blood cell, these plug-forming particles float in our blood vessels, looking for trouble. If they spot damage, they attach onto the injured blood vessel surface like burrs to dog fur. From that position they release a mess of proteins that sound the "I'm bleeding!" alarm. Other platelets then join in, like the paparazzi descending on Angelina Jolie, and form a holy huddle in an attempt to seal off the area. These micro-plugs act like crazy glue to prevent blood from leaking outside of our vascular walls. And they are very important. If we run low on platelet numbers, or if their function is lost, we can bleed spontaneously and die. But in cardiovascular medicine, having too few platelets, or ones that don't work properly, isn't the usual concern. The problem we face has more to do with too many clots and, in particular, ones in precarious locations. This is because platelets are programmed to play it strictly by the book. Any injury to a blood vessel gets a clot — no discussion and no exceptions. With this inability to select one type of blood vessel injury from another, platelets respond in a robot-like fashion to vascular injury, no matter if it's an annoying shaving nick or a critically narrowed heart artery. They respond by mechanically laying down a blood clot first and asking questions later. And if the clot is large enough, it can obstruct blood flow. Just like a beaver dam that sticks out into a running river, these blood clots can change the flow pattern in our arteries and, in some instances, stop flow altogether. To make matters worse, smoking enhances this blood-clotting process. Smoking cigarettes increases the stickiness of platelets, making them more likely to form bad clots. Since vascular disease is primarily a problem with clotting at the wrong time and place, we need to somehow rein in these platelets to prevent blood clots from jeopardizing our health.

Bring Out the Leeches

When looking for blood-thinning solutions, we don't have to go any further than our own backyard. That is, if your property backs onto a marsh or pond. The master of blood-clot prevention is none other than the leech. These cunning carnivores are specially equipped with all the tools to most efficiently remove blood from their hosts (innocent swimmers like you and me), and it's not just their nasty suction device that's at work. Leeches' saliva has three key ingredients that allow them to accomplish their dirty deed. First, these beasties produce a local anaesthetic that numbs our skin and allows them to avoid detection while they feast on our red blood cells. Out of sight, out of mind — until you come out of the water and see these black globs hanging off your naval. Second, their oral suckers release a chemical that dilates our blood vessels, like opening the beer spigot wide, increasing the flow of blood into their wide open mouths. Lastly, and most importantly to our discussion, they add a blood thinner to the mix. This third ingredient, called hirudin (pronounced "here-rude-in"), prevents blood from clotting, so the bloody heist remains uninterrupted for the twenty minutes or so it takes them to fill the tank.

Although these vampire wannabes, all slimy and gushy, disgust most of us, they have carved out an honourable place in medical history, nonetheless. For over two thousand years, leeches have been used for blood-letting. This was a popular medical procedure in ancient times, performed to rebalance the "humour" levels. Since most illnesses were thought to be caused by some disparity between your blood, phlegm, black bile, and yellow bile, it made sense at the time to remove the "excess" blood. Although the rationale for applying the leeches evolved somewhat over the years, their use increased steadily. Blood-letting was so fashionable in eighteenth-century Europe that its practice almost forced the wee monsters into extinction. Leeches were in such hot demand that local populations were decimated, necessitating the need for leech imports and even the development of leech farms as a major commercial industry. In the heyday of their use, it was claimed that leeches could cure anything from obesity and kidney disease to hemorrhoids and headaches. With little else to offer, applying leeches was a central practice for doctors, explaining why the word leech is so closely derived from the old English term for physician (*laece*). Any self-respecting medic needed a sure supply of leeches, and patients expected to have them applied, much as current patients expect an antibiotic prescription when they visit their GP with a sore throat.

Although it dropped off with the advent of improved medical therapies, the use of leeches in modern medicine has enjoyed a limited revival. Since the 1980s, surgeons have made use of leeches following reconstructive surgery. Because veins are difficult to surgically reconnect, blood can build up in the transplanted area and slow healing. Enter the leeches. For under $10 Canadian, hirudotherapy, as it's referred to, has been shown to double the success rate of skin-graft surgery. In cardiology we also make use of leeches ... well, indirectly. The leeches' blood thinner, hirudin, is a very powerful medicine to prevent blood clotting and is currently used for some heart attack patients as they recover. However, this type of blood thinner is not appropriate for preventative medicine, since no pill form exists, and the drug is just too powerful for our purposes. To help guard against unwanted blood clotting, we need a gentle poison, and preferably one that is devoid of blood-sucking creatures. So relax, no leeches will be recommended for use here.

Willow Bark's Welcome Bite

Willow bark has long been regarded as an important medicinal ingredient, initially because of its ability to treat fever, and, more recently, as an effective blood thinner that preferentially targets the blood-clotting platelets. As early as the fifth century B.C.E., Hippocrates, who is regarded as the father of medicine, included willow bark in his arsenal of therapies, alongside eye of newt and sweat of mule. He wrote about how to extract the bitter powder from the willow tree's bark and leaves, and how it could be used for relief of pain and treatment of fever. Before the nineteenth century's scientific era, medical research and development depended utterly and completely upon anecdotal trial and error. "It seemed to work for Great-Uncle Harry, so let's try it on you" was the prevailing wisdom. Considering the therapies of olden days, which included such unlikely ingredients as cat dung and dried semen, a trial is what they likely endured (for the poor patients), and error was the probable outcome. But while many such remedies were discarded over the centuries as useless or even harmful, willow bark remained prominently on the apothecary's shelf. The reliable benefit of willow bark was known early on in North America as well. Native Americans made use of it before Columbus's arrival on the shores of the new world, to treat headaches, fever, chills, sore muscles, and joint pain. The Reverend Edward Stone, a vicar from Oxfordshire, England, discovered this when visiting a Native settlement. He watched the medicine man at work and learned first-hand how they boiled the bark from the silvery white foliage over the open fire to make their elixir. In his diary entry from 1763 he recorded how effective the bark soup was in reducing fever in his afflicted settlers. For those interested in such natural therapies, dried willow bark is still available today and can be purchased in the form of powdered capsules or herbal tea bags.

In the late 1800s, physicians were caught up in a fever fad. Thermometers were included in the black bag tool kit and most practitioners used them obsessively since they viewed fever as the essential component of infection, rather than as a resultant symptom. They were concerned that fever would cause a patient's blood to coagulate and their tissues to burn up. So when the active ingredient from willow bark was isolated and found to reduce fever, it was a perfect case of supply meets demand. This fever-fighting active ingredient was called salicylic acid, and arrived on the market at the ideal time to fill the therapeutic needs of the hour. But there were some problems. The dose had to be worked out (again by trial and error), and something had to be done to reduce the nauseating, bitter taste and its unpleasant stomach irritation. A young chemist by the name of Felix Hoffman is credited for developing a less toxic form of the drug. Legend has it that his father suffered from rheumatism and was unable to tolerate the available formula because of tummy upset. So his boy took matters in hand and added a chapter to father-son bonding. Being facile with molecular manipulations, Felix was able to come up with a tamed version of salicylic acid that was named acetylsalicylic acid or ASA. By the turn of the nineteenth century ASA was a top seller. Today over 8 billion tablets are consumed in Canada each year. If only Felix could see us now!

Aspirin Comes of Age

The blood-thinning effect of Aspirin wasn't appreciated until after the fever fad had settled and the field of pharmacology matured. In 1948, Dr. Lawrence Craven, a GP from California, noticed that the patients in his practice who took Aspirin for their aches and pains seemed to be somehow protected from developing heart disease. But it wasn't until the early 1970s that the most important role of Aspirin was uncovered: Aspirin is platelet poison. In addition to relieving symptoms of fever and easing joint pain, Aspirin thins the blood by targeting the platelets specifically. It does this by attaching to receptors on the platelet surface, and prevents them from attaching to each other and clumping together. So with ASA on board, platelets spend their entire one-week lifespan alone in the world, with no other platelet to lean on for support. No platelet is an island. Having lost their ability to attach to each other because of Aspirin's therapeutic effect, platelets are less likely to loiter along the blood vessel walls, and blood clots are less likely to form. The key lesson for us is that Aspirin's blood-thinning effect dramatically reduces the risk of heart attacks and stroke.

In this scientific era of ours, the benefits of willow bark and its derivatives have not been left to anecdotal speculation. Aspirin has been extensively studied in recent years, in some of the largest scientific research projects to date. Studies have included people with heart disease as well as a great number of healthy volunteers, including doctors. Being good sports about science and posterity, physicians have signed themselves up over the years as guinea pigs for some of these studies to help establish Aspirin as a viable modern medicine. The U.S. Physicians' Health Study involved over 22,000 male doctors, who were followed for five years, to clarify Aspirin's relationship to heart attack rates.[1] When the results first came in, researchers were astounded and brought the study to an abrupt halt: Aspirin reduced the risk of heart disease by a whopping 44 percent. That means that those medics on Aspirin were two times more likely to skirt heart disease than their less fortunate colleagues taking the placebo sugar pill. The surviving docs were convinced by Aspirin's value and quickly started recommending it to their patients who were at risk for vascular disease.

But the predominately female nursing profession queried, "Is the advantage of Aspirin just a 'guy thing,' or can more sophisticated and highly evolved species also benefit?" They did their own study to see if ASA could also reduce heart disease in women. The Nurses' Health Study spanned six years and involved over 87,000 volunteer nurses.[2] Not surprisingly, the results were also favourable, showing that those women taking Aspirin had a lower incidence of heart attack, particularly those who were post-menopausal. These results paved the way for the Canadian Cardiovascular Society's recommendations in 1988 to replace *apple* with "an *Aspirin* a day to keep the doctor away."

To clarify the benefit of Aspirin with regard to stroke prevention, a group of researchers decided to lump together all the major population studies on Aspirin. The larger the scientific study, the more statistical power it has to answer the questions posed with greater certainty. One way to achieve this confidence is to compile like studies together into one larger study, a method called meta-analysis. The Antiplatelet Trialists' Collaboration is a group of Aspirin researchers that brought together all the Aspirin studies that had to do with cardiovascular risk reduction, to draw firmer conclusions about the drug's effects from a larger database of people.[3] Their meta-analysis was massive. With a patient sample of over 100,000 they were able to substantiate that Aspirin not only reduced the risk of heart disease, both in men and women, but also substantially reduced the risk of stroke. The bottom line was an overwhelming two thumbs up in favour of Aspirin use to reduce vascular disease — heart attacks and strokes.

However, not everyone has the same benefit with Aspirin. Those at the highest risk have the most to gain from taking their daily pill. If you smoke, your platelets are stickier and the risk of heart disease and stroke is higher. Aspirin helps to reduce this risk by "relaxing" those platelets. And nothing can work faster to reduce your risk. It takes as little as twenty minutes from the time you start chewing a regular ASA tablet for your platelet function to slow up. This is why the ER docs have patients with chest pain chew a couple of baby Aspirins on the spot. Time is of the essence. Even before the diagnostic tests have been done to define the cause of their symptoms, patients are asked to chew on ASA.[4] The drug can get to work right away if it turns out to be a heart attack and, if not, there is little harm in taking this small dose.

Between a Rock and a Hard Place

It was my intern apprenticeship year and I was covering the coronary care unit in the hospital for the first time. Overwhelmed by the responsibility and anticipating the worst, I prepared myself for a gruelling day's work by applying a double layer of Arrid Extra-Dry underarm deodorant and donning a clean pair of brown underwear. The casualty officer from the emergency room called up — "we've got an acute MI en route with a ten-minute ETA and will require lytic stat" (translation: "There is a heart attack patient on his way to our hospital, quickly approaching by ambulance. Please get your lazy butt downstairs here to help us make preparations, and bring some of that newfangled, clot-busting drug with you, pronto!"). So I did. The newfangled drug was called Streptokinase. It had just been approved for heart attack treatment and worked like Drano does on backed-up plumbing, digesting obstructing blood clots to re-establish normal blood flow to the heart muscle. I had read about the drug and had learned of the improved heart attack survival we could expect with its use. Opening a blocked heart blood vessel saves the heart muscle from being permanently damaged, which in some cases can mean the difference between life and death. But there is also a downside to these potent clot-buster drugs. As Spider-Man would say, "with great power, comes great responsibility." There's no way of directing the drug to the specific blocked artery in the heart. Once given, the drug circulates through the entire body looking for blood clots to destroy. Lacking any discrimination, they not only break down the bad clots that are messing with heart blood flow, but they can also dissolve the good blood clots, like the ones on the healing surface of a stomach ulcer or others holding blood from escaping from a wound. The most feared complication with using this type of medicine is bleeding into the brain. Fortunately, this happens in less than 1 percent of people receiving the drug, but when it does, it's always fatal. So there I was, holding in my sweaty hands this brand new wonder drug that had the potential to cure or kill. "Glad I'm under the dome," I thought.

I discussed the risks and benefits of the clot-buster with my patient, who was in the throes of a heart attack. "Sounds like a dangerous drug ... but what are my choices?" he asked, clutching his chest and gazing around the room at the heart monitor and emergency equipment.

"Fairly limited," I answered honestly. "If you don't want the medicine, then we'll have to take our chances with the heart attack. Some of your heart will be damaged, and that can cause trouble both now and in the long-term. If you agree to the medicine, then we'll have to take our chances with the possible side effects, like the bleeding issue we discussed. There's no guarantee that the medicine will successfully open the vessel, but it's the best we've got. Either way there are risks to take."

"Sounds like I'm damned if I do and damned if I don't," he surrendered, lying back onto the pillow and closing his eyes.

"Not quite," I countered in my best Dr. Kildare reassuring tone. "At least with the drug on board, there's a potential for benefit."

I had a similar discussion with the neurologist when I was wheeled into the trauma bay with my own stroke not so long ago. That time, it was me on the receiving end and my own life on the line. But either way, giving or receiving, such decisions can be challenging. And it's not always a happy ending. I survived, as did my patient, but we always need to weigh the benefits of any drug or procedure against its potential risks. Even our old friend over-the-counter Aspirin has the potential for side effects.

Any drug, whether prescription medication or over-the-counter herbal remedy, needs to be considered in your specific medical context. This is where your family doctor plays a key role. The doctor knows your medical history and can give a professional opinion on how the risks and benefits stack up in your specific case. Make an appointment and ask, "Any problems with me taking an Aspirin a day to help my ticker?" Besides, it's very important that your health care providers know that you're taking Aspirin. Some drugs can interact with Aspirin and may need adjustment.

Medications That Can Interact with Aspirin

- ACE inhibitors (such as Vasotec, Monopril, Prinivil, Zestril, Accupril, Altace, and Mavik)
- arthritis medications
- blood thinners (such as Coumadin, heparin)
- beta blockers (such as Tenormin, Lopressor, Corgard, Inderal)
- diuretics (water pills)
- diabetic medications
- acetazolamide (Diamox, for glaucoma)
- phenytoin sodium (Dilantin, anti-seizure drug)
- divalproex sodium (Depakote, anti-migraine)

The bleeding risk of Aspirin isn't anything like the clot-buster medicines, but it's not zero, either. Troubles typically occur when people with known bleeding problems or stomach ulcers take Aspirin to excess. Since ASA is broken down in the liver and removed by the kidneys, it should be avoided by people with significant liver or kidney disease. And because Aspirin is a blood thinner, your surgeon will want you free of the drug for a week before he puts you under the knife, since nobody wants post-op bleeding or a damaged reputation. I've been on daily Aspirin for years and haven't had any side effects with the drug or any issues of concern. But everyone's different and needs to weigh and balance the risks and benefits on an individual basis. Check out the list below to see how your risk/benefit equation looks for Aspirin and bring it up with your GP on your next visit.

Benefits of Aspirin	Risks of Aspirin
Reduced risk of heart attack	Upset stomach
Reduced risk of stroke	Heartburn
Fast action	Stomach ulcer
Simple once-a-day regimen	Increased bleeding risk
Inexpensive generic brands	Allergic rash

The Serendipity of Goldilocks

When you walk down the Aspirin aisle in your pharmacy you may be surprised about the choices presented. Forms of Aspirin include capsules, caplets, suppositories, and liquid elixir, available as brand-name products or generic no-name options. There's the standard adult 325 mg tablet, which you can get enteric-coated for tummy protection. If the regular dose isn't enough to dull your knee pain or headache, there's the 500 mg option, also in either tablet or capsule form. You can jazz things up a bit with flavoured Aspirin, cherry or orange (neither as good as the children's chewables from yesteryear). Women can get calcium-plus to supply that needed bone builder to the mix, and sugar-free Aspirin is available for those calorie-conscious folks wanting to avoid the corn starch binding additive in the regular tablet.

You may then ask, "Which dose of Aspirin is best to prevent vascular disease?" In the five largest studies looking at preventing heart disease (called "primary prevention"), the doses of Aspirin used varied from 75 mg once a day to 500 mg once a day. No single primary-prevention study to date has compared different doses of Aspirin to each other to see if one dose is better than another. But when platelet function is examined, 75 mg of Aspirin is enough to rein them in and help prevent vascular events. And since we generally want to take the smallest amount of any medicine to limit the side effects, going low makes sense.

"But then why are there only 81 mg tablets at the pharmacy, and no 75 mg tablets?" When I had a fever or headache as a child, Mom would give me some Aspirin, either as the medicinal chewing gum, Aspergum, or in the form of a candy-like, chewable tablet — an 81 mg tablet, a quarter of the size of an adult Aspirin. That was before we knew about Reye's syndrome. In the early 1960s, Dr. R. Douglas Reye and his Australian medical team documented a series of fatal brain-swelling cases in children. In the 1980s it was discovered that Aspirin could trigger such brain swelling if given to children suffering from a viral infection, like chicken pox. With the U.S. Surgeon General advisory in 1982, baby Aspirin was taken off the pediatric shelf. But before the ASA manufacturers dismantled their baby-medicine machinery, studies showing the benefits of low-dose Aspirin in preventing vascular disease started to surface. To meet the growing needs of the market, the pharmaceutical giants happily dusted off their baby Aspirin equipment, and have been cranking out the 81 mg tablets for vascular protection ever since. So the baby Bayer wasn't thrown out with the bathwater. There's no clinical difference between 75 mg of Aspirin available in Europe, and 81 mg available made in North America. Like Goldilocks and the three bears, we want a dose of Aspirin that's not too much and not too little, but just right. And the baby Bayer is just so.

Ingredients for Supplement Soup

Not everyone can tolerate Aspirin, even the baby-coated kind, and some just prefer to get back to the bark and take a more natural remedy. Alternative, or complementary medicine, is very popular. It's reported that over 50 percent of the Canadian population takes some form of alternative medication, whether it's garlic to lower cholesterol or echinacea to stall the common cold. The rapidly growing billion-dollar industry of herbal remedies owes some of its success to the general discontent many have with mainstream medicine. Molière said that "doctors pour drugs of which they know little, to cure diseases of which they know less, into patients of whom they know nothing." But our current understanding of pharmacology is more sophisticated than ever before, and rigorous research efforts are continually refining our understanding of the interactions medications have in our bodies. Contrary to popular belief, there is no big-book-of-stuff-that-doctors-know-but-don't-want-to-tell-you. Many of our current therapies derive from plant sources, and mainstream medicine is very interested in botanical ingredients that may indeed be a valuable resource for future medicines.

My mother-in-law loves to bring out her box of German and Asian herbals, a cure for everything. She and others are under the illusion that the term "natural" implies safety. I try to gently remind her that although water is natural, it is the most common cause of drowning. So just because some remedies have natural origins, it doesn't mean they're risk-free. Although my comments often get lost in translation with her, it remains important to realize that using alternative medicines can lead to trouble. Similar to the potential problems with prescription drugs, alternative therapies can also produce adverse drug interactions and cause side effects. For example, St. John's Wort, used by some to improve mood, causes a serious interaction with anaesthetic agents, dangerously lowering blood pressure during surgery. As well, 180 dietary supplements have the potential to interact with warfarin, a common blood thinner, and more than 120 alternative therapies, including high-dose vitamin E, alfalfa, and coenzyme Q10 can interact with Aspirin. This underscores the need to let your MD and your pharmacist know everything that you're taking, so troubles can be avoided.

Use of alternative therapies may play a valuable role in managing a variety of ailments, particularly when recommended by health professionals, but because this arena is rife with charlatans, caution is needed. In 1861, a so-called doctor, C.V. Girard, advertised that his ginger brandy drink was "a certain cure for cholera, colic, cramps, chills, fever … and a delightful and healthy beverage." Reading the labels of alternative therapies today, you'll still see broad claims of cure. But further investigation will disappointingly demonstrate a distinct lack of scientific evidence — often none at all. Unlike the Himalayan heaps of scientific literature undergirding Aspirin as a premier preventative medicine, no such data exist for the alternatives. As well, herbals aren't under the same quality-control scrutiny as prescription medications and therefore have no verifiable claim with respect to their safety and efficacy. This lack of standardization among alternative products means that just because the label says ginseng, doesn't guarantee that it is pure or guarantee how much you're actually getting. One scientific study profiled in the *Lancet* medical journal rang the fraud alarm by analyzing fifty brand names of commercial ginseng.[5] They found that all of the products sampled had less than 10 percent of the active ingredient, with six of the samples devoid of any (one ginseng product even contained the decongestant ephedrine, not advertised on the label). Some reliable websites to check out before you make any herbal investments include www.familydoctor.org and www.quackwatch.com. Talk to your family doctor or pharmacist for advice about the alternative therapies you are taking and their quality.

The Essential Omega-3

For the longest time the cardiology community was strictly recommending a diet low in fat. Dr. Dean Ornish's low-fat approach was proven effective in reducing plaque buildup on heart arteries and still stands as an important contribution for heart-disease prevention. However, while it is true that some fats, most commonly saturated doughnut-pastry-poutine types of fat, are indeed harmful and should be avoided like platform shoes or a red-stained parachute on sale for half price, we've come to realize the significant benefit of other fats for our cardiovascular health. Omega-3 fatty acids are a good example. The name *omega-3* comes from the description of its molecular structure, which is really only important to the undergraduate student of organic chemistry, the night before the final exam. More useful to know is that omega-3 fat is an *essential* fat. Our bodies can't produce it but they need it to function properly. Therefore, it's *essential* that we have omega-3 somewhere on our grocery list.

The discovery that certain fats are essential dates back to the 1930s, in the heydays of rat experimentation. Rats who subsisted on a fat-free diet were quick to develop problems with growth, reproduction, kidney function, even scaly skin (a real social stigmatizer for the appearance-sensitive rats), all of which vanished like magic when their cooks added back fat to their rodent recipes. Human population studies supplied the next level of evidence supporting the benefits of certain dietary fats.[6] Our brothers and sisters in the land of the midnight sun added significantly to these data. Historically, the Inuit diet has revolved almost entirely around fish, and in the past their rates of heart attack or stroke were the lowest in our fair land. (Unfortunately, that's all changed with the northern migration of fast food.) Fatty fish, like the ones able to survive Arctic Ocean conditions, are packed full of omega-3 fatty acids and this helps to explain why those who eat more fish have fewer heart troubles. Over the past thirty years, there have been over 7,000 scientific reports published to examine the role of essential fat in our diets, and thousands of clinical trials on the heart benefits — and in people, not just rodents.

The two types of essential fatty acids are omega-3 and omega-6 fatty acids, but it is only the omega-3 variety that carries the heart health benefit. Unfortunately, most of our North American diets are high in the omega-6 type and low in the omega-3. So to help reduce the risk of heart attack and stroke, we need to reverse this dietary bias. Exactly how omega-3 fat protects the heart is still on the agenda for discussion, but one of the key benefits has to do with its blood-thinning role. Omega-3 fat reduces our blood-clotting capacity, and this may very well explain the significant reduction in heart attack rates that is documented in those groups who have higher intakes of this essential fat in their diets.

The best source of omega-3 fatty acids is seafood. The Canadian Cardiovascular Society suggests eating two fish meals per week to supply our hearts with the ideal amount of omega-3 fatty acids.[7] There are two main biologically active products in omega-3 fat: EPA (eicosapentaenoic acid) and DHA (docosahexaenoic acid). Fatty fish like mackerel, lake trout, herring, sardines, albacore tuna, and salmon are high in both EPA and DHA.

Sources of Essential Fatty Acids

- fatty fish, shellfish
- walnuts
- flaxseed (linseed)
- canola oil, soya oil
- pumpkin, sunflower, chia seeds

Other dietary sources include various nuts and seeds. These plant-derived forms are converted in the body from linoleic acid to omega-3, but not in a consistent fashion. For a reliable dietary source of essential fatty acids, it's still best to eat fish.

"What about omega-3 eggs?" you ask. Well, it's a bit of a gimmick, for sure, and certainly not nature's way. Omega-3 concentrations in eggs are achieved by feeding chickens flaxseed, which isn't part of their ordinary diet (I'm told that the chickens don't really like the flaxseed, so you end up getting a thin-shelled egg of discontent). These eggs are somewhat more expensive, and the only way you get the omega-3 part is by eating the yolk, which you should know is high in bad cholesterol (300 mg, or a week's allowance), offsetting the advantage of the value-added egg. You're probably better off to eat the flaxseed on its own, ground up and sprinkled over your morning cereal, and to buy free-range eggs from your local farmer for a heart-healthy, egg-white breakfast omelette.

If you're serious about getting your essential fat from botanical sources, corner a dietician. They are the experts when it comes to practical food choices to achieve the maximum health benefits. Your family doctor can set you up with an appointment to discuss these and other dietary issues with one of our valued professionals. In the meantime, check out Canada's Food Guide online (www.hc-sc.gc.ca) under the Food and Nutrition option, or the www.dieticians.ca website.

You hate fish, you say? Fish oil, containing omega-3 fatty acids, is one of the best natural products available. But the hardest part of shopping for any supplement is finding one you can trust, with the active ingredients you want. Supplements don't have to follow the same rigour as medications, and can vary wildly in terms of quality. It's buyer beware, so take care! The labels have the amounts of EPA and DHA listed. You want to choose the omega-3 product with quality amounts of both EPA and DHA that has been purified to remove environmental toxins, particularly mercury. Your pharmacist can steer you to the better supplement choices and away from the scams. But, remember, supplements, like all medicines, have a potential for side effects. The downside of omega-3 supplements is that they tend to have a fishy aftertaste, and they can cause some tummy upset. That's not all. At high doses (over three grams per day), omega-3 capsules can raise cholesterol and blood-sugar levels, and increase your tendency to bleed. If you do decide to add them to your daily routine, include them on your list of medications so your family doctor is in the loop. For supplement takers, the recommended dose is 1 to 2 grams per day. If you're on Aspirin already, I would keep it to only 1 gram a day of omega-3.

Mad About Fish

I hated fish as a kid. Growing up in landlocked Ontario was not a good location for developing an appreciation for fresh seafood. When Mom would call us for dinner with the words, "fish is ready," my siblings and I would drag our heels, knowing that greasy, little, battered smelts were waiting to be de-boned. It wasn't until I moved to the West Coast in my teens that I discovered the miracle of barbecued salmon and halibut. And it's in this form — the naturally packaged form — that I prefer to get my omega-3 fatty acids (I'm one of those pesky pesco-vegetarians). I eat an average of two meals of fish per week, which supplies not only the essential fat my blood vessels need, but is a high-quality protein source, and particularly tasty, especially if you choose wild Pacific salmon, barbecued on a cedar plank, with freshly squeezed lemon, a sprinkle of cilantro …

"Well, what about mercury poisoning? Aren't you worried about the heavy metal content in fish?" I'm asked, usually by prairie folk who are just looking for another excuse to eat more triple A beef.

"Not worried as much as disappointed," I reply.

Just when eating fish has been shown to be beneficial for the heart, along come industrial pollutants to spoil the show, giving people licence to return to fast-food hangouts. And where was this mercury scare about bioaccumulation in fish when I was a kid, being force-fed battered smelts? I would've loved to have used that excuse on my parents — "Sorry, Mom, I'd really like to finish my plate of fish, but you know … mercury levels and all. Can you pass the fries, please?"

In Lewis Carroll's *Alice in Wonderland*, the hat-making host of the tea party was portrayed as demented for good reason: hat-making was hazardous to the brain. In the mid-1800s, beaver felt hats were all the rage in Europe, likely the reason Canada got a rodent as its national symbol (and not something more dignified like an elk or moose). To shape the hats into the desired fashion, the hat-makers used hot solutions of mercuric nitrate. They typically worked in poorly ventilated spaces, thereby ensuring a generous and all too often toxic exposure to mercury. Hatters of the time commonly suffered from slurred speech, tremors, irritability, shyness, depression, and other neurological symptoms — summarized in the expression "mad as a hatter."

But even in modern times, mercury poisoning is serious business. The largest recorded case occurred in the late 1960s from the release of methyl mercury into the sea near Minamata, Japan, killing over a thousand people and disabling many times more. The reason that fish contain high levels of mercury is due to a phenomenon called bioaccumulation. Mercury settles into the water vegetation, small fish eat it up, medium-sized fish eat them, and large fish ingest it all. Bioaccumulation in the aquatic food chain magnifies the exposure. So the old, large, predatory fish get the high mercury levels building up in their bodies, landing on your dinner plate. In the early 1970s, Health Canada established a guideline level of 0.5 ppm (parts per million) for mercury in most commercial fish. The fish with levels of mercury that exceed this safety maximum include shark, swordfish, king mackerel, tilefish, as well as fresh and frozen tuna, supporting the Canadian Health advisory to limit meals of these gourmet fish to once per week, and only once per month for women of childbearing age and children. Fortunately, none of these are particularly common here in Alberta, and none are on my favourites list. Other contaminants, such as PCBs (polychlorinated biphenyls), can be minimized by removing the skin and trimming the fat from the fish, but the mercury gets stored tightly in the flesh and organs, so you can't cut it away. Not all fish are heavy on the heavy metals. Salmon, canned tuna, and shrimp generally have lower levels of mercury and would be good examples of seafood to add to the weekly menu. There is no evidence that moderate consumption of these types of fish in Canada poses a significant health hazard, indicating that we can have our fish cake and eat it, too.

Peter's Prescription

My patient, Peter, is at high risk for having a heart attack or stroke. After reviewing the Framingham Risk Score results with Peter and his daughter, I recommended a baby Aspirin daily to help reduce his risk for vascular disease. Even though you can buy it over the counter, I wrote out a prescription for enteric-coated ASA 81 mg, to make it official.

"I prefer to take Tylenol when I have aches and pains," he argued.

"That's fine," I said. "Go right ahead. But acetominophen [Tylenol] won't protect you from heart trouble the way ASA can," I stressed. In preventative cardiology, it's the platelets we're trying to dull, not the pain fibres.

"Well, sometimes I use Advil, too. That's like Aspirin, isn't it?" Peter questioned.

"Yes, both are inflammation fighters," I granted, "but only Aspirin knocks out the platelets the way we want. The non-steroidal anti-inflammatory drugs, or NSAIDs like Advil, don't thin the blood as effectively. Taken with Aspirin, NSAIDs increase the risk of tummy irritation, ulcer formation, and bleeding. And since they share similarities with Aspirin, they tend to compete with it and can reduce Aspirin's effectiveness to do the blood-thinning job. If I were you, I'd take Tylenol for pain and avoid the NSAIDs altogether."

"What about Plavix ... the super Aspirin that I've heard about at school? Would that be even better for Dad to take than regular Aspirin?" asked Peter's daughter, clearly keeping up on her pharmacology reading.

Impressed, I replied, "I suppose ... if you can afford it." Clopidogrel [Plavix] costs big dollars, Aspirin just pennies. I don't recommend the super Aspirin unless someone has a heart attack or stroke while taking regular Aspirin. If Aspirin alone isn't effective in preventing vascular issues, then using more expensive meds like clopidogrel is certainly warranted. Not everyone responds to ASA and may need a more powerful agent for protection. "I don't think this is a job for super Aspirin," I said, smiling. "Let's start with regular ASA, one a day to keep disease away, and on our next get together, I'll review some other ways you can reduce your risks."

DEFENDING THE LINING

Smoke Screen

Since I last saw Peter and his daughter, he had been reviewed by a lung specialist to check out the damage he had done with all those years of smoking. As is routine, a copy of the consultation letter was sent to me to keep me in the loop. His daughter asked if she could see it, so I passed them the letter. She read it aloud as I took Peter's blood pressure. Here's an excerpt:

> "Mr. H. has smoked a total of 36 years starting in the year 1971 at the age of 15, on average a half of one package per day, a total of 18 pack years (36 years x 1/2 pack), approximately 6,570 packages of cigarettes or 164,250 individual cigarettes. Various studies have reported that smoking one cigarette on average will shorten the smoker's life expectancy from six to eleven minutes. Therefore, smoking may have shortened Mr.

H's life expectancy by as many as 1,255 days or about *3 years.* This does not include morbidity from smoking related illnesses occurring prior to death."

"Did you find that helpful?" I asked, somewhat embarrassed that one of my colleagues would communicate in such aloof statistical-speak.

"Not really. I mean I already knew that smoking was hard on my health. The detailed math doesn't help me. Besides, what's it matter if I kick off when I'm ninety years old instead of ninety-three?" Peter asked, smirking.

"Now that's wishful thinking if I've ever heard it," I said, grinning. "I suppose losing your last three years when you're all grey and shrivelled in a nursing home doesn't sound all that bad. However, the number crunching of this letter is only a commentary on your health risks as they specifically relate to smoking. The letter's forecast doesn't take into account your *overall* risk of heart disease that we calculated with the Framingham Risk Score. With your particular risk profile, there are more than just three years at stake. But no need to get too morbid here or bogged down in numbers. It's time for a picture." I pulled out a sheet of blank paper and grabbed one of my many shirt pens to make a sketch. "I'd like to give you a visual. I call this the PLAC diagram. My hope is that it might give you a clearer indication of where we need to go to reduce your risk of heart disease ... while you quit smoking, of course."

PLAC Attack

The picture I penned for Peter and his daughter is a simplified cartoon and is supposed to look like a blood vessel cut in cross-section. I chose this vantage point to illustrate the main layers of our blood vessel wall. Smoking does a number on each of these layers, and we need to counter those insults if we're going to keep the blood flowing freely and the

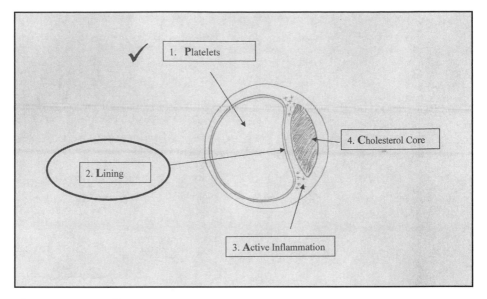

Figure 3.1: PLAC diagram.

heart beating happily. The central hole in the blood vessel is called the *lumen* (pronounced "loo-men"). I drew it askew, not because I had too much coffee to drink, but to include a vascular plaque in the wall of the artery. This type of plaque shouldn't be confused with the tartar around our gum line that dentists love to pick at. Vascular plaques are fat deposits that develop within the walls of our blood vessels in response to years of hard living. They sit there behind the scenes and increase in size slowly as our middle-age years pass, and are the major cause of heart attacks and stroke. Most Canadian adults have them brewing in their arteries, ready to raise Cain at the first opportunity. Our goal is to limit these opportunities. To do this we need to bolster our vascular defences at four key places in our blood vessels.

The acronym PLAC stands for: Platelets (the blood-clotting cells that flow through the central hole of the vessel); Lining (the innermost layer that protects the wall from the clotting blood); Active inflammation, indicated by the little x marks, that occurs within the wall of the vessel making it more prone to disease; and the dark shaded Cholesterol Core that builds up deep within the vessel wall and can distort the central hole as it grows, reducing the flow of blood. With this diagram in hand I outlined these four anatomical areas for Peter and his daughter. Since we'd already discussed the need for blood thinning, I put a check mark beside Platelets.

"Let's move our attention to the blood vessel lining," I said as I circled Lining. "This Saran Wrap layer, lining the inside of our blood vessel wall, is a critical line of defence against atherosclerosis attack. To reduce our risk of heart disease, we need to protect this lining as a top priority."

Such discussion of "lines of defence and attack" always throws me back into some old Second World War movie memory, usually one with John Wayne swaggering out of a muddy trench, yelling to his troops to "move it out!" The analogy between heart disease, as played out on the surface of our blood vessels, and trench warfare is striking. We may not be aware of the battle, but it rages daily in our blood vessels, creating more casualties than any other disease process. To reduce our risk of being one of these casualties, we need to bolster our defences. Consider the French Maginot Line, built along the border between France and Germany. It was designed to keep out the advancing Nazis, and was believed by many to be impenetrable. But despite its elaborate fortifications, the wall failed in the end, when the Nazis cleverly moved their offence *around* the barricade. Our vascular ramparts are similar. They can handle a certain amount of action, but a breach of defence is inevitable if the attack persists and the line remains unsupported. If we want to prevent plaques from getting a foothold, and thwart the efforts of heart disease and stroke, we'll need to consider sending in some reinforcements to defend our Maginot lining.

Rice Paper Walk

Not to downplay John Wayne's dominating presence on the silver screen, but I'm a bigger fan of David Carradine. As in *Kill Bill*, his roles are more complex and unpredictable. My favourite Carradine character is Kwai Chang Caine, the fugitive monk, in the TV series *Kung Fu*. I recently rented one of the early episodes for my boys, and they've been throwing karate chops and roundhouses at each other ever since. In addition to imitating the fighting scenes, they were particularly fascinated by the various tests the young apprentice was given by his religious teachers. As you may recall, to graduate, the grasshopper, had to prove his speed by snatching a coin from his master's hand, to show his pain tolerance by carrying the red-hot cauldron with his forearms across the room, and finally to prove his deftness by walking across the rice paper floor without leaving a mark.

The innermost lining of our blood vessels is like this rice paper floor. It's called the endothelium ("endo" meaning "inner," and "thelium" meaning "wall"). This lining is made of a single layer of cells, and covers the inside of all our blood vessels, from stem to stern. Measuring only one one-hundreth of a millimetre in thickness, it's many times thinner than Carradine's rice paper, but has to withstand a lifetime of hard knocks, such as, for example, inhaled cigarette smoke. This microscopic barrier keeps the continual torrent of blood, which flows from our pumping hearts through to the smallest capillaries, from clogging our arteries. Without this intact lining, our blood cells would instantly stick to our blood vessel walls, and flow would come to a standstill — as would we. Like the disapproving glance from the grand master at poor Kwai Chang's dented rice paper, any mark on our blood vessel surface represents a failure of our cardiovascular health. Injury to our vascular lining gives the green light to vascular plaques. Once these injuries start to establish themselves, heart attack and stroke aren't far behind. To reduce our risk of atherosclerosis (the buildup of vascular plaques) we need to protect this critical lining, ASAP.

Elevated pressure inside our blood vessels is an all too common cause of damage to our rice paper vascular lining. Like trying to bike uphill and into the wind, high blood pressure makes it harder for our lining cells to do their work. If the pressure doesn't let up, soon the lining does, and plaques develop. Consistently elevated blood

Defending the Lining

pressure damages the artery walls and turns the surface from slippery to sticky. And the last thing we want — even less than receiving a tax audit or watching MuchMusic — is a sticky blood vessel surface. Our circulating platelets can't help themselves. They see damaged lining, and they say "hello blood clot."

How Tall Is Your Blood Pressure?

The measurement of blood pressure dates back to the early colonial era, before the rash of red, white, and blue flags popped up south of the border. The credit goes to the Reverend Stephen Hale, a curious clergyman who carried out a rather messy experiment on his horse — don't try this at home! In 1733, when Vicar Hale was sipping his heavily taxed English blend with perhaps too much time on his hands and not enough complaining parishioners, his thoughts veered from high church to high blood pressure. He spied his old mare put out to field and thought, "I wonder if it be possible to measure blood pressure using a glass tube attached to the neck artery?" He couldn't leave such a provocative question unanswered. So, much to the chagrin of his horse and without the SPCA to intervene, the right and good reverend tied down old Nellie and began the historic experiment. Wanting to avoid his cup from running over, he chose a glass tube nine feet in length, calibrated for easy measurement. With the help of his stable boy and a copy of *Horse Anatomy Made Ridiculously Simple* he inserted a brass beer spigot into the horse's neck artery (that's the messy bit). To the spigot he attached his Goliath-sized glass tube, held vertical by his hired hand, who was perched precariously on a stepladder. When all was in place, he opened the spigot and watched as the horse's bright red blood bubbled up the glass tube, reaching, as he recorded for posterity, the eight-foot three-inch mark. Although variations on Hale's experiment were repeated by surgeons performing leg amputations during the American Civil War, the technique never really caught on as a clinical standard — just too darn messy, I guess.

Over the following years various non-invasive devices were developed to estimate blood pressure indirectly, avoiding the Monty Python paint-the-town-red, blood-spurting dilemmas. Initially, wrist and finger devices were marketed, but weren't found to be very accurate. In 1905, a Russian surgeon by the name of Nicolai Korotkoff discovered that he could hear blood pressure if he tied a tourniquet around a patient's arm and listened with his stethoscope. This listening, or auscultation, method proved to be most accurate at estimating blood pressure without the muss and fuss of inserting tubes into arteries. Modern digital readout blood pressure machines are based on the same methods used in those one-hundred-year-old antiques. As they do today, the early gadgets used a column of mercury as a pressure reference, calibrated in millimetres of mercury (mmHg), rather than in feet and inches. Since mercury is nearly fourteen times denser than water, the column needs to be only about a foot high and can sit unobtrusively in the clinic office. If it were a water column it would have to be the height of Reverend Hale's tall tube, and would stretch well through the ceiling of my office.

Since high blood pressure doesn't produce symptoms, and is often referred to as the silent killer, one of the challenges is convincing patients to take their pills to lower it. I've sometimes wondered if it would be more convincing to report blood pressure in terms of feet and inches of water, rather than in millimetres of mercury. "You really should take these pills, ma'am. You may only stand five foot two, but your blood pressure is over eight feet tall!" And with every incremental increase in blood pressure, our lifespan shortens. Modifying Robert Frost's observation that "happiness makes up in height for what it lacks in length," it could be said of high blood pressure that "hypertension makes up in height for the years it lacks in length." To help reduce injury to our blood vessel lining, the shorter the blood pressure the better.

Pressure Cooker

Although doctors have been able to measure and document blood pressure for many years, its clinical significance wasn't appreciated until more recent times. Take the case of the former U.S. President Franklin Delano Roosevelt as an example. His medical record painfully illustrates that we have to do more than merely measure and document blood pressure. We have to control it.

In 1935, at the age of fifty-three, FDR was entering his first term as president. His medical record indicated that his blood pressure measured in the high normal range of 135/85 mmHg. But by 1940, with the ever-present weight of leadership on his shoulders, doctors noted that his blood pressure had climbed to 170/90 mmHg. Today this would sound the red alert, but in that era of vascular pre-enlightenment his doctors dutifully noted the measurement in their charts and carried on with their day — golf, perhaps. And, as with most things gone bad, like fish forgotten in the fridge, time generally only makes them worse. By 1942, months after Germany declared war on the United States and while FDR was mired in Midway and the internment of Japanese Americans, his blood pressure had climbed to a dizzying 180/105 mmHg. He was advised to rest — advice which he did follow, while he continued to chain-smoke. In 1944, with declining health following his fourth and final election, his blood pressure was a critical 205/120 mmHg. In 1945, while sitting for a portrait in the White House, he complained suddenly of a terrific headache. Hours later, he was dead, diagnosed with a fatal stroke from a burst blood vessel in his brain. At the age of sixty-three, one of the most beloved of American leaders was felled by elevated blood pressure — a death easily preventable today.

High blood pressure is one of the common insults to our blood vessel lining. About 25 percent of our population, which is about twice that of Toronto, has elevated blood pressure. On a world scale, high blood pressure is a major contender as a cause of premature death. It ranks as the third leading cause, just behind smoking and malnutrition. And it's not all about death and dying. High blood pressure causes scores of illnesses, from kidney failure and eye damage, to limb loss and impotence (another kind of "limb loss"). If blood pressure is left untreated, the risk of having a heart attack or stroke increases two to three times. Despite this realization, high blood pressure doesn't get recognized enough. Of the 8.3 million Canadians with high blood pressure, over 40 percent of them are unaware of the silent killer they harbour, and are carrying on, oblivious to the serious and growing risks it has for our health.[1] To protect our vascular lining we need to ensure our blood pressure gets measured and is kept well under control.

Wrinkles in Time

My three-year-old son is still in the edible stage of cuteness. I love to play with his supple little face, pull his ears, and squish his forehead to resemble Worf, the Klingon from *Star Trek*. His skin is so pliable that he doesn't even seem to notice, until one of his brothers brings my kibitzing to his attention and he swats me away. What makes his skin so malleable is its composition. The skin of youth has elastic fibres that give it that springy stretch and recoil resilience. The cosmetic industry has invested untold millions to discover its secret (to sell at a premium to the aging populace). But alas, no such cure for aging skin has been discovered. The scores of products that sit on the shelves of beauty salons, each claiming to be able to turn back the hands of time, do little more than provide a mask behind which to age. "Have no fear, Botox is here!" beauticians counter. This nerve poison gets rid of wrinkles, sure. By paralyzing the facial muscles, Botox flattens out the wrinkles. But it does nothing to return a youthful complexion. Movie stars may look a bit younger from a distance, but directors don't want them on camera: paralyzed facial muscles make for flat expressions and dull performances. Youth is gone. Suck it up, Cher.

As we move past our twenties and thirties, the elastic fibres in our skin are systematically and continually replaced by collagen protein. This replacement is hardy enough and able to stand up to the knocks life dishes out, but it lacks the suppleness of our yesteryears. Instead of youthful stretching and recoiling, older skin just stretches and stays stretched. So now, when you smile, it's the hard-etched lines around the mouth that show themselves prominently, perhaps accentuated by a double chin and an assortment of crow's feet. But it's not just our skin that's aging, *all* of our connective tissue age this way — the "Dici or nothing" days are done. And this predictable aging effect is true for our blood vessel walls as well, and is the most common cause of high blood pressure.

High Expectations

Blood pressure is on the rise in Canada. With us boomers hitting middle age and beyond, high blood pressure is reaching epidemic proportions in our society. While less than 10 percent of young adults, thirty and under, have hypertension, the numbers rise to over 50 percent by the time we hit freedom fifty-five. That means that if you bought the debut album by The Doors, your chance of having elevated blood pressure is in the 50/50 range. So now it's not just about "Mr. Mojo rising" anymore. Better get that pressure under control, before "this is the end."

This predictable increase in blood pressure with aging has to do with the loss of elastic stretch in our blood vessels. When the heart pumps blood into circulation, the walls of our blood vessels take the hit. The elastic fibres in the walls of our arteries act like shock absorbers. And like a good running shoe that absorbs the brunt of the road — so our tender tootsies don't get too tender — our blood vessels take the load. They do this by going with the flow and expanding to accommodate the wave of pumped blood. This stretching of our muscular arteries allows the increased pressure that the heart generates to be absorbed into the wall, and prevents the smaller arteries downstream from feeling the full force of the heart's contraction. But, as we age, the elastic response of these large arteries falls off. Like old runners that have seen one too many 10K fundraisers, our artery walls don't absorb the impact all that well. Rather, the stiffened walls pass the buck onto the smaller arteries down the line. These smaller calibre vessels weren't designed to handle this kind of pressure. Repeated over and over again, numbering more than 100,000 beats per day, 24/7, this sledgehammering on our small blood vessels damages their lining. Plaques form as a response to this repeated offence, and permanent damage to our kidneys, heart, and brain inevitably follows.[2]

This loss of youthful, arterial stretch is why blood pressure increases quite predictably as we celebrate our fiftieth birthday (although it doesn't help when a large group jumps out from behind sofas yelling "surprise!"). Twenty percent of the Canadian population has high blood pressure or hypertension, and every year the number gets bigger. Most of us will become part of this statistic. Our lifetime risk of developing elevated blood pressure exceeds 90 percent. And no, smoking won't help. Some claim to feel more relaxed after a drag, but the nicotine in a cigarette increases the heart rate and, at least temporarily, increases blood pressure. If anything, the combination of smoking and aging spells added trouble for the lining of our blood vessels. So while you quit, we need to sit hard on elevated blood pressure to reduce the ongoing damage to our blood vessels.

Why So High?

"Why is it that so many of us have high blood pressure?" you may be wondering. Let's face it, 8.3 million Canadians is a lot of people! The list of potential causes is a long one and, like most lists, dreary to review. But most of the items on the inventory are uncommon, including several rare glandular disorders that are difficult to pronounce, unless you did a minor in classics. The vast majority of people with elevated blood pressure get the moniker essential hypertension. In doctor-speak, it means that we essentially have no easy answer to "why so high?" Genetics likely play a role, as does the aging of the population, but neither can entirely explain the epidemic proportion of hypertensives crowding the clinics. The common denominator for most people with elevated blood pressure is living in our North American culture: stressing about their jobs, eating salty fast foods, sitting in front of a computer screen all day, drinking too much alcohol, and self-medicating with anti-inflammatory pills.

Regardless of the level of hypertension, the best approach to lowering it is to take a hard look at how physically active we are, and at what we eat and drink. This list includes some of the main players that heighten blood pressure.

What Heightens Blood Pressure?

- psychological stress
- high salt intake (beyond 2,400 mg/day or 1 teaspoon)
- sedentary behaviour (expect 5–10 mmHg higher if sitting all day)
- weight gain (expect 5 mmHg for every 5 kg excess fat on board)
- alcohol in excess (three or more drinks per day increases BP)
- over-the-counter anti-inflammatory (e.g., Advil)

In our pill-popping era, where any problem, from performance anxiety to hyperactivity, is considered best solved by medication, we tend to only glance at these lifestyle interventions and pay them casual lip-service. But unless we incorporate these manoeuvres into our day-to-day activities, blood pressure rises, in spite of medications we take. If we want to reduce the damaging effect of high blood pressure on our circulatory system, we will need to address all of these so-called lifestyle catalysts.

How High Is High?

The first time I had my blood pressure measured was by a fellow student in a St. John Ambulance first aid class. I was surprised how tight the cuff got during the procedure and startled my nervous classmate when I let out a shriek. What I didn't realize at the time was that the pressure in the arm cuff had to be high enough to stop the flow of blood in my arm temporarily. When blood pressure is measured, two numbers are reported: the first represents the amount of pressure inside your arteries when your heart is contracting, and is referred to as the systolic pressure. The Greek word for contraction is *systole* (pronounced "sis-tollee"). The second number is the diastolic pressure, correlating to the pressure in our system when the heart is in diastole (pronounced "die-ass-tollee") or relaxed mode. Traditionally, blood pressure is notated like a fraction, with the systolic number on top of the diastolic, with the units "millimetres of mercury" assumed (abbreviated as mmHg). So for example, a normal blood pressure would be stated as 120/80 mmHg.

Blood pressure is considered high when it exceeds an accepted threshold, and medics use the term hypertension to provide a diagnosis for those who have elevated blood pressure. The blood pressure level that defines hypertension is getting lower as we learn more about the devastating effects of elevated pressure on our cardiovascular system. Currently, we use 140 millimetres of mercury as the systolic cut point to separate those with high blood pressure from those with normal pressure. Classification schemes have been developed to categorize patients according to blood pressure severity.

Blood Pressure Classification

Blood Pressure Category	Top Number (systolic BP mmHg)	Action
Normal	< 120	Good, but let's keep it low.
Pre-Hypertension	120–140	Not so good. Dietary factors needed.
Stage 1	140–160	Bad. See your doctor this month.
Stage 2	> 160	Ugly. See your doctor this week (ideally tomorrow).

Such classification methods allow physicians to identify which patients are at highest risk for blood pressure trouble.[3] Having a threshold number like 140 mmHg has helped to simplify treatment strategies and allowed us to sort patients into study groups to advance our understanding of heart disease. However, such a black-and-white approach can be misleading and may have oversimplified the problem of high blood pressure, giving many a false sense of reassurance. Any threshold number is an arbitrary line. Sure, a group of world-class experts gathered, they drank pots of coffee, ate stale Danishes, and agreed upon a number. And, yes, their decision to choose 140 mmHg as the cut point for hypertension was based on a massive amount of data detailing the relationship between high blood pressure and heart disease. But the problem with this algorithm approach is that it doesn't follow the ways of nature. Biology isn't all-or-none. High blood pressure increases the risk of vascular disease in a continuous fashion. There is no magic number, past which "bing," you're in trouble, and under which "whew," you're safe. The health risks associated with high blood pressure increase steadily as the pressure rises, millimetre by millimetre. Half of those with pre-hypertension (defined as a systolic pressure between 120 and 140 mmHg) will develop hypertension, with its attendant troubles, within four years, unless they make lifestyle changes.

This relationship between increasing blood pressure and the concomitant increased risk of vascular disease is illustrated in these graphs. The systolic blood pressure numbers are plotted on the left-hand graph, and the diastolic numbers are plotted on the right-hand graph. On each graph, patients are divided into age groups that span a decade, to show the relationship between aging and blood pressure problems. What we see is that the risk of stroke goes up steadily from a systolic pressure of 115 mmHg in a smooth line as the pressure increases. When we examine the data in detail, we see that there is no evidence of a magic threshold number. Regardless of the age group, this linear relationship holds true: the higher the blood pressure, the greater the likelihood of trouble.

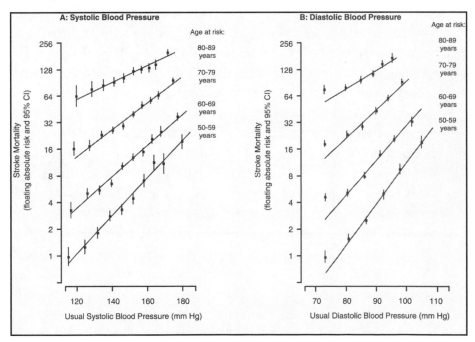

Figure 3.2: Rising blood pressure and rising risk. S. Lewington, et al., "Age-Specific Relevance of Usual Blood Pressure to Vascular Mortality: A Meta-Analysis of Individual Data for One Million Adults in 61 Prospective Studies." Lancet 360(9349) (December 14, 2002): 1903–13.

So, if you go into the local drugstore and check your pressure (which I think is a really good idea about now), don't think that a top number under 140 mmHg necessarily means you should light up to celebrate. We need to work towards keeping our pressures as low as we can for the long haul. Go to your local drugstore and get your blood pressure checked. Record the number and share it with your family doctor on your next visit. Managing blood pressure is like playing golf; the lower the score the better the game.

Why I Don't Wear Plaid and Paisley

Most of my patients have elevated blood pressure when I check them in my office for the first time. This is partly because hypertension is a common condition seen in the cardiologist's office. But also it's because patients are often quite nervous, and the mercury reading will climb upwards when we're anxious. Our blood vessels respond to a litany of environmental cues, including time of day, visual images, temperature swings, noise, and, of course, being freaked out in the doctor's office. It is well known that white coats evoke an emotional response of tension and panic. This white-coat hypertension may be responsible for some of the elevated blood pressure readings observed in the cold, cruel, sterile settings of medical clinics. For this reason most of my colleagues leave the white lab coat at the hospital, and we don our civvies when we see our outpatients. As well, to promote calm and relaxation, we take considerable care in choosing serene colour schemes when designing our office spaces. We purposely stay clear of the bright primary colours used in fast food restaurants that scream, "hurry up and eat so more people can come in and spend their money on our low-quality, fatty food."

Blood pressure can vary by 20 to 30 mmHg over the course of the day. It's typically higher in the early waking hours when our stress hormones are being pumped out, to help us deal with imminent bad coffee and inevitable heavy traffic on the way to work. Body position and activity can also affect the readings. Blood pressure increases when we cross our legs or if we're talking during the measurement, and it can fall when we rise from a lying position. As well, there is a certain degree of error in blood pressure determination, in part related to equipment limitations and the skill of the practitioner. This is why we need to take a series of measurements, using appropriately sized arm cuffs and calibrated machines. Before we make a diagnosis of hypertension, we measure the blood pressure serially, usually over a number of separate visits, with the patient quietly relaxed. Making the diagnosis can sometimes be difficult. For challenging cases, we make use of a twenty-four-hour blood pressure monitor, which measures blood pressure at prescribed intervals while the patient is at home and participating in regular activities of daily living. Such a day-in-the-life-of-blood-pressure record has been shown to improve diagnostic accuracy considerably.

I encourage my patients to have their blood pressure checked in their local drugstore, away from the paramedic panic or, better yet, to purchase their own equipment allowing them to measure their blood pressure in the quiet and comfort of their own home. Digital monitors can be purchased at your local department store or pharmacy and cost between $60 and $100. The Canadian Hypertension Society website (www.hypertension.ca) lists the blood pressure devices currently approved, and your pharmacist or family doctor can check your device to ensure that it's measuring correctly. To improve the accuracy, it's best to have your blood pressure checked at the same time of the day, twice a day, morning and evening. The average blood pressure is more important than any isolated reading. A simple approach is to take five measurements over the course of the week. If your device doesn't store the numbers, write them down in a journal and discard the highest and the lowest values, or *outliers* as they're called, and then average the remaining three. These home readings are valuable to share with your family doctor and will make it easier to arrive at the proper diagnosis and allow for most appropriate treatment options to be considered.

Salt of the Earth

My earliest memory of salt isn't so much the taste; it's the large, wooden salt boxes on the roadside that I recall. Motorists used to scoop it onto the icy streets to make them more passable. In fact, salt was so liberally used on our local roads in Ontario that our Ford Maverick nearly fell apart from corrosion over just two winters. Despite its corrosive effects on metal, salt is the premier preservative, with applications dating back to before recorded time. Since salt draws out moisture and prevents decay, the ancient Egyptians used natron, a salt mixture, to mummify their departed royalty. Even more valuable than creating morbid museum artifacts was the use of salt in the food industry. Historians consider food preservation as one of the critical foundations for civilization, and salt has been featured prominently on this front since antiquity. In ancient Greece, salt was a valuable commodity, commonly used in the slave trade, giving rise to the idiom "being worth your salt." The Romans used salt like money, and our word *salary* comes from the salt ration paid to Roman soldiers.

My aunt from "the old country" used to pickle everything. It was how they managed, eking out an existence without preservatives, like potassium sorbate, sodium benzoate, and, of course, refrigeration. By using a salt-water brine, perishable food can be kept for months at a time. Despite living in our chemical stabilization age, she continued to store dozens upon dozens of jars in her pantry, including the conventional sauerkraut and cucumbers, as well as pumpkin, peppers, beets, eggs, pork, meatloaf, onions, jalapeños, cauliflower florettes, a variety of olives, and even watermelon rinds. When we came over for a meal, we would sit down to a regular salt feast. True to the studies of children that have illustrated the preferences of the young palate for salty foods over sour or bitter, my siblings and I loved it. Chowing down on my aunt's salty fare was no issue for me as a child. Young, supple blood vessels can readily accommodate the extra fluid that salt sequesters. But when you crack fifty and push into "middle youth," the care-free, salt-scarfing party is over. This innocent-looking white granular crystal, which has found its way onto every dining table in the country alongside our processed food, is the single most common cause of high blood pressure in North America.

Salt Content of Some Foods

1 serving ham (100 g)	1,000 mg
Canned soup	800–1,200 mg
1 dill pickle	1,500 mg
1 cup sauerkraut	1,500 mg
Processed meats	ten times more than fresh meat

Reasoning for Less Seasoning

The American Medical Association made a statement recently about the need to reduce sodium content in processed food by 50 percent to help control the hypertension epidemic.[4] Not low enough in my opinion, but it would be a start in the right direction to begin to rein in the food industry. They estimated that if salt consumption were cut down by 1,200 milligrams a day, there would be 20 percent fewer people with high blood pressure and 150,000 lives saved each year, from sea to shining sea. Canadian cuisine is no less salty, and the importance of salt restriction is just as important north of the forty-ninth parallel.

So the obvious thing to do is to avoid salty foods, but in our high salt environment, this means doing more than just giving up the gherkins. Dieticians tell us that we need to keep our daily salt intake under one teaspoon, or 2,400 milligrams.[5] The problem is we don't measure out dietary salt this way. We add a dash here, and eat a bag of potato chips there, and consume great quantities hidden away in processed foods. Following an all-too-common diet of bacon (727 mg for two slices) and sesame bagel (540 mg) for breakfast, chicken noodle soup (850 mg) with a ham submarine sandwich (1,210 mg) for lunch, and a slice of pepperoni pizza (1,445 mg) with a side of barbecue-flavored potato chips (213 mg) for dinner, it's easy to pass the one-teaspoon mark several times over (according to my calculations, that works out to 4,985 mg of sodium, which is over twice the recommended daily intake).

The first step in reducing salt intake is to clear the table of any source of salt. If you find yourself in "Margaritaville, searchin' for some lost shaker of salt," don't look too hard. Added salt is the surest way to overdo it on the salt loading. And it's not just the obvious little glass salt shakers — you also need to lose the soy and teriyaki sauces and ditch the condiment tray. Most spreads and condiments, including ketchup, mustard, and relish, offer too much in the salt department for those of us concerned about blood pressure. Salt substitutes may have a limited role here. The majority contain potassium chloride instead of salt's sodium chloride (even the "no salt" products, like Mrs. Dash have some potassium in the mix). Potassium chloride makes for an obvious salt substitute for two reasons: first, it tastes like salt, since it's the chloride ions that our taste buds notice, not so much the potassium; and second, it doesn't bind to water as sodium chloride does, so our blood pressure gets a break. Although studies have shown that blood pressure can be lowered using potassium substitutes instead of regular salt, adding potassium liberally to food can cause other problems, particularly if the kidneys aren't working at peak function (check out the perils of hyperkalemia on Wikipedia). And then there's the bitter metallic taste of such products, and the theoretical concern about radioactive exposure from the beta-gamma emitter potassium-40 (K-40) present in most salt substitutes. It's been said that the error of youth is to believe that intelligence is a substitute for experience; while the error of age is to believe experience is a substitute for intelligence. Generally, I'm not a fan of substitutes — the real McCoy or nothing, thanks!

The second logical step to reduce salt is to eat mostly foods that don't contain much and to avoid those that do. The Dietary Approach to Stop Hypertension study, better known by the acronym DASH, showed that dietary choices can make an important difference in blood pressure control.[6] The classic experiment involved 459 hypertensive adults divided into two groups: one to follow a diet rich in fruits and vegetables, with low-fat dairy products and items with reduced saturated fat; and the second group following a typical U.S. diet. At the beginning of the study and after two months, the blood pressures in both groups were measured and compared, and the people following the DASH diet had a significant drop in blood pressure. Details about the diet are on the Web (www.heartandstroke.com under the subheading "Eating Well"), and if you're interested, a DASH Diet sample menu is listed below. One way to get around the heavy use of salt in your cooking is to experiment with some recipes that use a variety of herbs and spices, like fresh garlic, lemon juice, flavoured vinegar, cumin, nutmeg, cinnamon, tarragon, oregano, and good old fresh-ground pepper.

The DASH Diet Sample Menu
based on 2,000 calories/day

Food	Amount	Servings Provided
Breakfast		
orange juice	6 oz	1 fruit
1% low fat milk	8 oz (1 C)	1 dairy
cornflakes (with 1 tsp sugar)	1 C	2 grains
banana	1 medium	1 fruit
whole wheat bread (with 1 Tbsp jelly)	1 slice	1 grain
soft margarine	1 tsp	1 fat
Lunch		
chicken salad	¾ C	1 poultry
pita bread	1/2, large	1 grain
raw vegetable medley:		1 vegetable
carrot & celery sticks	3–4 sticks	
radishes	2	

loose-leaf lettuce	2 leaves	
part skim mozzarella cheese	1.5 slice	1 dairy
1% low fat milk	(1.5 oz)	1 dairy
fruit cocktail in 8 oz (1 C) light syrup	1 fruit	½ C
Dinner		
herbed baked cod	3 oz	1 fish
scallion rice	1 C	2 grains
steamed broccoli	½ C	1 vegetable
stewed tomatoes	½ C	1 vegetable
spinach salad:		1 vegetable
raw spinach	½ C	
cherry tomatoes	2	
cucumber	2 slices	
light Italian salad dressing	1 Tbsp	½ fat
whole wheat dinner roll	1 small	1 grain
soft margarine	1 tsp	1 fat
melon balls	½ C	1 fruit
Snacks		
dried apricots	1 oz (1/4 C)	1 fruit
mini-pretzels	1 oz (3/4 C)	1 grain
mixed nuts	1.5 oz (1/3 C)	1 nuts
diet ginger ale	12 oz	0

Figure 3.3: DASH Diet sample menu. Courtesy of L.J. Appel, et al., "A Clinical Trial of the Effects of Dietary Patterns on Blood Pressure." DASH Collaborative Research Group. *New England Journal of Medicine* 336(16) (April 17, 1997): 1117–24. See www.nih.gov/news/pr/apr97/Dash.htm.

I know for many, diet is a four-letter word. Generally, those who make a passion of their diet often expect too much from their food choices. Diet is not a panacea to cure all ills. But the opposite is also true: those who pay no attention to their diet expect too little in terms of health benefit from their food choices. I'm not a diet fan myself, but I do see some value in understanding nutritional underpinnings, especially when it comes to controlling blood pressure. The DASH diet diverges from the typical North American diet primarily in its lower fat content, with use of low-fat dairy products, for example, and its emphasis on fresh fruit and vegetables. So rather than needing to meticulously follow the DASH diet rules and regulations, we can get the bulk of the benefits by making dietary adjustments in the produce department. Besides, we're not talking about trying a temporary diet to lose weight for an upcoming grad reunion. Ours is a long-term health strategy to make sustainable improvements in blood pressure control.

When it comes to eating, it's easier to add than subtract. Instead of considering all the foods you need to cut out to lower salt, think rather about all the options you can add in. If you add in fruit and vegetables at every meal and snack, you will leave less room for salty fare. For example, my daily routine looks like this: I start with my morning banana and granola; then there's the mid-morning apple before my coffee break; at lunch, I eat a generous portion of pre-cut carrot sticks with my sandwich; and then for the mid-afternoon, half a grapefruit with a handful of soy nuts; the late afternoon tub of cut vegetables; and finally, the dinner salad with my evening meal. This approach easily satisfies Canada's Food Guide's recommended five to twelve daily servings of fruit and vegetables and keeps my salt exposure to a minimum. This way, I'm never hungry and I'm always getting the low-salt nutrition my blood pressure needs to keep it under control.

Salt Mine Scenarios

In ancient Rome, and more recently in Stalinist Russia, a spell in the salt mines was the fate of dissidents and criminals. In our high-salt society, it's the fate of every Canadian, once you leave the safety of your own home. For instance, I find it hard to avoid salt loading when I'm at a movie. Fortunately, in this home entertainment/DVD day and age, we don't frequent movie theatres as often as in the past. But when I do, it's nearly impossible to steer clear of the salt, with that pervasive odour of fresh, buttery popcorn filling the air. So to limit the damage, I choose the small popcorn. I know for just twenty-five cents more I can get a medium, but I just don't need the salt, not to mention the empty, butter-loaded calories. No matter which size of popcorn you buy, you're going to finish it completely, so you might as well buy the smallest amount and temper that mindless eating reflex that we go into once we're passively fixed on the movie screen with the all-encompassing THX sound — "the audience is listening" to be sure, and scarfing down popcorn as well.

Eating out at a restaurant can also be a tricky place to limit salt ingestion, especially if you're in celebration mode. I don't want to be a killjoy, but with a few pointers (five in total), I'm sure you'll be able to enjoy yourself without overindulging on the salty side of life.

- Before the meal, put the salt shakers, soy sauce bottle, and condiment tray on someone else's table, lest you be tempted.
- When ordering an aperitif, check out the wine list first. If choosing a highball, avoid the Caesar or anything else containing tomato juice.
- If you have a hankering for an appetizer, avoid the battered salty types like Buffalo wings or deep-fried calamari. Veggie tray (minus the dip) is your best choice. Ask for a low-salt soup.
- When you're considering your entree avoid the obvious salty picks containing cured or smoked meats, like ham or sausage, processed cheese, pickles, anchovies, or olives. Search for the freshest options. Ask about the specials; they're the ones that the chef is going to take most pride in and prepare best, with likely the least amount

of salt added. Beware of items with loads of extra seasonings, like super-spicy Cajun halibut. If their fish requires such spices to be served, it's probably older than you want, and they're trying to get rid of it before it evolves into a legged creature and walks out on its own.

- Ask your server to put all sauces, including gravy and salad dressings, in a bowl on the side. This way you can use less without compromising the intended taste. Heavy sauces cover a thousand sins in the kitchen. The freshest ingredients are healthiest and require the least doctoring. I avoid sauces, dressings, and gravies and prefer unadulterated food, with perhaps a dash of pepper.

A Stitch in Time — Skip the Brine

Since we generally get 80 percent of our sodium intake from processed foods and at restaurant meals, we also need to be salt-aware as we go grocery shopping. My six-year-old looked up at the wall of sweet cereals. "Why is all the food that tastes good, bad for you, and all the yucky stuff healthy?" he asked, as we were grocery shopping together. "I think that's what the food companies want you to think," I replied. "That's why they package their products so brightly with cool pictures and stack them at the head of each aisle so everyone sees them when they first come in. They make their money from this packaged and processed stuff, but it's full of sugar, fat, and salt, and not very good for our bodies. No one makes much money from good, old-fashioned goodness, like fresh apples, so they're just piled off to the side in the hopes that we choose the corn chips and cookies instead," I said, pushing the cart over to the produce section. "Well, how about you get the apples for you and this for me," he smiled, holding up a giant bag of Frito Corn Chips.

The best approach to grocery shopping without packing on the salt is to leave the kids with a sitter and make a mad dash to the perimeter of the store. For the most part, you'll be safest away from the wasteland of the aisles. Fill your basket with fruit, vegetables, and low-fat dairy products. With the exceptions of the cooking staples, like canola oil, whole wheat flour, and the like, there's limited value in the aisles, lots of expensive convenience packaging, and far too much salt. Addition of salt is an industry standard for food processing. Check out the labels, which now indicate the percentage of daily intake per serving (a magnifying glass may be required here for the fine print). Dieticians suggest avoiding products with more than 10 percent of our daily salt requirements. And beware: the food manufacturing industry is always trying to sneak their products under the health radar. For example, don't be fooled by terms such as *reduced salt* or *light in sodium* plastered over the packaging, since these adjectives refer to *comparably* less salt. Soy sauce, for example, is a high-salt choice, no matter if it's touted as having *less* sodium or not. It's like saying Alexander the Great was less of a tyrant than Genghis Khan. Let's face it, they both had significant adjustment issues, and neither is going to cut it as a school trustee or church deacon. And there's more! Labels like *unsalted* and *no added salt* don't mean salt-free. Peanuts, canned vegetables, butter, and microwave popcorn are all examples of salty foods labelled in this manner. This clever branding simply means that no salt was added to the item during processing.

Fresh food is always better than processed. You get vitamins, minerals, fibre — all in a natural, easily absorbed form, the way nature intended it. Unless you're preparing for impending disaster, you don't really need canned anything. So if it's processed, put it back on the shelf. When you purchase processed foods, your hard-earned, post-tax dollars are being spent on the processing and packaging of the food, not the nutrition. Processing oftentimes removes nutrients. For example, enriched flour is simply the adding back of thiamine, niacin, folate, and iron, which are lost during flour processing. By avoiding processed foodstuffs you will be saving cash and reducing dietary salt, all in one fell swoop. If you must opt for a processed food item, better to look for the sodium-free or salt-free options.

Last Call

Mark Twain quipped, "Everything in moderation … including, of course, moderation." And sure, it's important to mark the important moments, let our hair down, laugh out loud, and paint the town red. I don't mean to be a wet blanket, but on the topic of alcohol consumption, moderation really is the best approach for optimizing the health benefits derived from alcohol, while reducing the risks.[7] We physicians are all quite eager to make mention of the various scientific studies lauding the benefits of red wine, especially as the bartender is taking orders. There are significant theoretical grounds for imbibing one or two drinks — good cholesterol rises, inflammation decreases, and insulin sensitivity improves. There is even data showing that moderate alcohol consumption is better than abstinence for reducing cardiovascular risk. But few of us swirl and sip with these benefits in mind. We enjoy the social lubricant alcohol provides, dulling us to the boring company and dreary discussions. But as soon as the threshold of moderation is crossed, any benefit of alcohol quickly falls away. Alcohol in excess is associated with an extensive litany of health hazards, ranging from liver cirrhosis to breast cancer. My medical textbooks would have been substantially thinner and easier to tote around, had alcohol never been added to the list of evils we do in the dark. And this is without including the staggering insults alcohol has had on our social landscape: marital strain, family abuse, domestic violence, and motor vehicle accidents often involve alcohol prominently in the mix.

Thanks to fallen celebrity icons like John Belushi emblazoned in our minds, we are generally aware of the lethal implications of drug overdose. Alcohol is no different and has claimed many lives, famous and infamous alike. The optimal dose for cardiovascular benefit is about 15 grams. This is roughly one to two drinks per day. The type of alcohol doesn't matter so much — cocktail, high ball (1.5 oz), beer (12 fl oz), wine (6 oz) — it's the amount of *alcohol* that's the issue, not the amount of fluid, colour, texture, bouquet, nose, finish, hint of chocolate, or flutter of strawberry. When it comes to hypertension, consumption beyond the 15 gram point causes blood pressure to rise in a predictable fashion. If you wake up with a hangover, you've crossed the line from medicinal benefit to overdoing it. So when the server informs you that it's "last call," remember the wise words of Ringo and say, "no, no, no, no, I don't drink it no more, I'm tired of waking up on the floor," and call it a night.

Of course, alcohol isn't the only beverage that, if taken to excess, can raise blood pressure (see Figure 3.3). The coffee craze has vaulted caffeine towards the top of the list of culprits, but it's not actually the coffee that's to blame — it's the caffeine in the coffee. And it's not just the java hunters who need to be concerned. Caffeine has found its way into a wide variety of products, from chocolate bars, soda pop, and so-called energy drinks to most over-the-counter drugs. Somewhere between 80 and 90 percent of us consume caffeine in some form or another on a daily basis, with most of us getting over 300 mg a day. It's a useful exercise to read the labels and see how much of this pep drug has been added. Caffeine reduction can help to keep blood pressure in check.

Caffeine Dietary Sources	Example	Serving Size	Caffeine
Cola	Coca-Cola Classic	355 ml (12 oz)	34.5 mg
Chocolate	Hershey's Special Dark	1 bar	31 mg
Energy Drink	Red Bull	250 ml (8 oz)	80 mg
Tea	Orange Pekoe	250 ml (8 oz)	50 mg
Coffee	Regular	250 ml (8 oz)	100 mg
Coffee	Starbucks Venti	625 ml (20 oz)	500 mg

Peter's Pressure

To help reduce the white-coat phenomenon, patients in our clinic have their blood pressure measured while they relax in a quiet consultation room. We use an automated cuff that takes three pressure measurements over a ten-minute period. This way we can record an average blood pressure before any white coat even enters the room. Peter's systolic blood pressure readings were elevated: 146, 148, and 152, averaging out at 149 mmHg.

"We need to get that blood pressure of yours down," I said. "Your blood pressure numbers are high, and you have evidence of heart muscle thickening on your electrocardiogram. This means your heart has to work harder than it should to squeeze out the blood. I suggest we use a medicine that can bring things under control in short order."

"Oh, I hate taking pills," Peter mumbled under his breath. "Isn't there anything else I can do?"

"Well, you could try acupuncture," I said. "It's been shown to help reduce blood pressure. Mind you, the folks in the study who benefited had to have regular needling four times a week, for thirty minutes a session. Such an approach to blood pressure control is generally felt to be a tad expensive and time-consuming for most."

Peter grimaced in agreement.

"Will Dad have to take medication forever, or is it just to get his pressure down?" his daughter questioned.

I smiled. "Forever is a long time to consider. Most people with high blood pressure need two medicines to keep it under control. And since blood pressure tends to go up as we age … if anything, your dad may require a number of medicines to control his blood pressure in the future. Cutting back on the salt will help a great deal, but generally, if medicines are needed to control blood pressure now, they'll likely always be needed."

I gave Peter his prescription with a "med sheet" to start him off with a personal medical record.

He sighed. "It's going to be tough to remember to take it every day."

"Well, you have no problem remembering to light up. What is it, sixteen times a day? Why don't you keep the pill bottle next to your smokes at night, and then in the morning when you go for your first nicotine fix, your blood pressure pill will be waiting for you," I suggested, with tongue in cheek.

Example of a Medication Record

Medication	Dose	Timing	Concerns
ASA	81mg	daily	Bleeding risk
ramipril	5 mg	daily	Dry cough

4

YOU SNOOZE OR YOU LOSE

Confessions from the Bedroom

Peter complained of being tired when I asked how he was feeling at our next appointment. I didn't expect the blood pressure medicine to be at fault. Although almost any drug can produce almost any side effect if you look hard enough, the medication I chose to help control Peter's blood pressure has only very rarely been reported to cause fatigue. I asked him about his sleep pattern, wondering if perhaps he struggled with lack of sleep, like the majority of Canadians.

"Sleep?" Peter shrugged. "No, I don't think I have any trouble with sleep."

"Maybe not for you," his daughter interrupted. "But the rest of us suffer. He snores like a chainsaw! Mom sometimes has to leave the room and sleep on the guest bed. And none of us got any sleep when we were camping in the tent trailer together. That's why Barb and I used to pitch the tent," she confessed to her father. And to me, she said, "We even sang him a Helen Reddy song with the words changed to 'I'm a snorer, hear me snore' for his last birthday." She giggled.

I smiled politely, but glancing at my watch, inwardly hoped I wouldn't have to hear a rendition.

"Yeah, that's true," Peter agreed. "And my wife has told me that sometimes she gets scared that I stop breathing. Sometimes she wakes me up in the night and tells me that I need a kick-start once in a while." He rubbed his ribs.

"Do you take naps during the day?" I pressed further.

"If I get the chance," he said, "I try to sneak in a catnap most days, and have zero problem falling asleep."

"That's for sure," his daughter added. "You even fell asleep reading to us at night when we were kids."

"Lack of restorative sleep can cause daytime fatigue and sleepiness," I said. "And what's more, insufficient sleep can lead to damaged blood vessel lining. It's stressful for our body when we don't get enough sleep. Stress hormones impair the normal functioning of our blood vessels. We've got your blood pressure under control. Now we need to address your lack of beauty rest."

Angelic Ascent

Unsatisfied with his cuddle-cub toy, our three-year-old still wants my company when he's trying to relax to sleep. A self-declared Ferber-failure, I consistently cave in to his pleas for a bedfellow. After our routine of story and prayer, I turn on the night light by his bed, press "play" to start the lullaby music, and cuddle up next to him until he's asleep. On the occasional evenings that I don't drift off first, I have the opportunity to watch him go to sleep. As with most children, once the bogeyman has been given his walking papers, sleep comes quickly. There's a bit of fidgeting and tossing and turning, but he soon settles into a position of comfort and happily doses off. The first thing that I notice to confirm my son's sleeping state is that the muscles of his arms, legs, and face begin to relax, punctuated by slight, jerking motions of his arms or legs. Of the five stages of sleep, this drowsiness correlates with sleep's first stage. Experts in sleep study define the various stages from light to deep by measuring brain-wave activity.[1] This is accomplished by placing electrodes on the scalp and recording the electrical activity, using an electroencephalogram, or EEG, but I have yet to resort to such technology at home.

Sleep Stages	EEG Waveform	Characteristics
Stage 1	transition from alpha waves (8–12 hertz) to theta waves (4–7 hertz)	light or drowsy sleep sudden muscular twitches can occur
Stage 2	theta waves (3–6 hertz) with bursts of sleep spindles (12–16 hertz) (a burst of brainwave activity visible on the EEG, signifying stage two, deeper sleep)	light sleep reduced muscular activity complete loss of awareness
Stage 3	delta waves (0.5–4 hertz) begin to occur	deep or slow wave sleep sleepwalking and sleep-talking behaviour can occur
Stage 4	delta waves (0.5–4 hertz) occupy over half of waveforms	deeper version of stage 3
Stage 5	EEG is similar to awake state with alpha and beta waves (8–30 hertz)	rapid eye movement (REM) vivid dreaming

Stage one is light sleep; if I try to get off his bed at this point, my son awakens easily and grabs onto my neck with a reprimand not to leave. So I settle in again and wait for him to drift into the deeper realms of sleep, when brain activity slows further and stirring is less likely. Very soon I'll notice his breathing is slower and more pronounced as he goes deeper. It's difficult to wake him once he's entered this deep sleep stage. I can wrestle my arm from under his head, rise from the creaky bed, and even inadvertently knock the tape player off the night stand, and he sleeps on, as I successfully sneak out of the room. It's during the deep sleep stages that some people sleepwalk and children may experience bedwetting (we've kept a plastic cover over the mattress just in case). But I don't always make scarce when my son nods off into the never-never land of sleep. If I do decide to linger, after about twenty minutes I'll notice that his eyelids start to flit and flicker. This signals the onset of the so-called rapid eye movement, or REM, sleep. Now I know he's truly entered dreamland, and I take my leave to do the same.

Sleep is a far cry from the absence of activity. It's a busy bit of physiology that involves a consistent internal structuring of the five sleep stages, which together comprise a sleep cycle. Following a well-organized temporal sequence, each sleep cycle, from the beginning of stage one to the end of REM, takes about an hour and a half to complete. During sound sleep, most of us will repeat the sleep cycle four to five times before the alarm goes off and the snooze button takes the hit for our late-night television viewing. Nighttime awakenings typically occur when we complete one sleep cycle and begin to re-enter the light stages of the next. This is when a snoring spouse, the tick-tocking of a grandfather clock, or a full bladder is more likely to grab attention and allow our consciousness to surface. Not all of the stages of sleep are the same duration. About half of our time asleep is spent in the deeper stages, and about one-fifth in REM sleep. Although there is also some dreaming during the non-REM sleep stages, more vivid dreams occur during REM sleep. As the night wears on, more time is spent in REM sleep, for a total of about two hours in adults, explaining why we're more apt to remember a dream first thing in the morning. Dreaming aside, both REM and deep sleep are essential parts of the normal sleep cycle, each contributing to the night's success in restoring our body's heart and soul.

The Importance of Zeeing Ernest

Birds do it, bees do it; everybody sleeps and has to, for health's sake. Without sleep our life expectancy is reduced to about ten days. In fact, all through the animal kingdom, sleep makes the shortlist for essential activities. Money and sharks may not partake, but sleep is as critical to the survival of us Homo sapiens as food, shelter, and reproduction. Why this is the case is under speculation and, despite all our fancy machines and know how, our need for sleep may never be fully clarified. While much about sleep remains a mystery to us, investigations have consistently shown that restorative sleep plays a central role in a wide variety of functions, from the intellectual arena of problem-solving ability and memory consolidation, to the physical realm of muscle growth, hormonal balance, and the maintenance of our immune system.

Our cardiovascular system also needs proper amounts of quality sleep for optimal function. When we sleep, we enter a hibernation-like state: our heart rate and respiration slow, blood pressure falls, and body core temperature drops. Since the workload for our heart is directly related to both the heart rate and blood pressure, slumber brings a relative reprieve for our incessantly pumping hearts. But the benefits of sleep for the heart are more deep-seated than mere energy management. Sleep brings restoration to our heart and vessels, without which the day's damages can develop into disease.

Unlike the ground squirrel and hedgehog that hibernate to wait out the winter, we remain rousable from our sleep-induced stupor and make use of this metabolic slowing, not so much to conserve energy, but to divert energies to the tasks of repair. It is during our sleeping hours that the lining of our vasculature is revitalized. The

You Snooze or You Lose

injuries suffered by our blood vessel linings from the day's combat, like smoking that pack of cancer sticks, eating the double chocolate doughnut, and arguing during the staff meeting, are repaired by the work of specialized, white blood cells, filling in the potholes and smoothing out the bumps while we sleep. What's more, sleep gives our vascular cells an opportunity to reinforce their armour in preparation for another day of cellular battle. The cells that make up our vascular lining produce nitric oxide, which functions to protect our blood vessels from the wear and tear of daily stressors. As we dream, nitric oxide stores are replenished and make our vascular lining less susceptible to injury. If you smoke, this is a crucial issue, since smoking disrupts deep sleep at night and depletes nitric oxide supplies during the day, rendering our blood vessels even more susceptible to injury. Habitual, sound sleep restores levels of this protector to normal, optimizing vascular health and reducing the risks of vascular disease, while you quit.

"Every Breath You Take, I'll Be Watching You"

The first recorded case of sleep-disordered breathing dates back to Greek mythology, in the story of Ondine's curse. It's a sordid tale of fatal attraction, spite, and adultery, but, nonetheless, nicely illustrates some of the potential health risks that can arise at the sleep/breathing interface. My understanding is that Ondine was a water nymph with a penchant for hot tubs and carousing with the mortals. She was bored with the primped and preened offerings of Mount Olympus and preferred mortal flesh. Smitten by her charm, one of her human lovers made a hasty oath that his "every waking breath would be a testimony of his love." He should have stressed, of course, that he meant this as a poetic metaphor, not to be taken literally, because when she caught him messing around town she totally lost it, cursing that if he should fall asleep, he would forget to breathe. And despite an all-nighter, with excellent Lamaze breathing technique, he eventually did fall asleep from sheer exhaustion, and his breathing did stop. The moral of the story: playing the field can take your breath away.

Breathing-disordered sleep is a common health problem, affecting approximately one-quarter of Canadian men and nearly 10 percent of women between the ages of thirty and sixty years. Peter's symptoms of daytime somnolence and fatigue, combined with his heavy snoring and interposed breathing gaps, are suggestive of a sleep disorder called obstructive sleep apnea. Middle-aged, overweight men are the prime targets for this condition, but it can affect anyone. Excess oral tissue obstructs the windpipe during sleep when the mouth is relaxed. This disrupts airflow, causing the loud snoring. Occasionally the oral tissue can completely obstruct air flow and temporarily stop respiration. These episodes can be scary for the bed partner, left in the uncomfortable predicament of waiting for the next breath to come. And like counting steamboats after a lightning flash, the bed partner is greeted by a thunderous snort, signalling the return of breathing. This period of "no breathing" is referred to as *apnea* ("pnea" is breath and "a" is none-at-all). During these apneic episodes, when breathing is obstructed completely, blood oxygen levels plummet, and the metabolic waste product, carbon dioxide, builds up. But, thankfully, patients with sleep apnea don't share Ondine's curse. When the carbon dioxide levels reach a certain threshold, their bodies wake them up, to allow for needed breathing. One may not awaken fully to recall the event, but just enough to gasp in a sleepy stupor, until gas exchange of oxygen for carbon dioxide is brought back to normal. This broken sleep cycle is often repeated throughout the night, explaining why such patients are tired all the time and able to sleep at the drop of a hat. Many affected don't even realize they've got a problem, and oftentimes it's the poor, sleep-deprived spouse who brings it to medical attention.

Treatments for sleep apnea are available to greatly improve sleep patterns and reduce daytime fatigue. Some people have improved sleep if they position themselves on their sides instead of flat on the back, so their oral tissue doesn't as easily obstruct windpipe airflow. Most people's sleep apnea will improve with weight loss so there's less soft tissue pushing on the windpipe. If it is medically indicated, some will benefit by wearing a breathing apparatus that props open the air passages while they sleep. Strengthening the upper airway muscles can also help, and I understand that in Australia, some people with sleep apnea find relief by playing the Australian drone pipe, didgeridoo (but with all that droning, who can sleep?).

My primary interest in sleep is in its relationship to heart disease. Untreated, obstructive sleep apnea is associated with a 70 percent increased risk of heart disease.[2] Prolonged and repetitive obstruction of breathing places enormous strain on our cardiovascular system. During these apneic episodes, blood pressure skyrockets, heart rate accelerates, and stress hormones, including adrenalin and cortisol, are released into circulation. Over time, these stress hormones directly damage the lining of our blood vessels, accelerating the atherosclerosis process. As well, chronic elevation of cortisol reduces the ability to sleep and creates a downward spiral of sleep deprivation, adding to the vascular stress.[3, 4] The good news is that treatment of sleep apnea not only improves airflow and beauty rest, but remedies vascular function, reducing the risk of heart attack and stroke.

Stolen Slumber

I was at a cardiology conference recently and made the mistake of signing up for a particularly dull afternoon program. Being with a group, I couldn't exactly skip out, although the thought repeatedly crossed my mind as I strained to stay focused. To help prop my eyelids open, I decided to grab a coffee during the afternoon break — it was only 2:00 p.m., after all — lots of time for the caffeine to wear off before bed. It's a rare moment of weakness when I let the baked goods at Starbucks attract me, but because of the long line-up at the till, the temptation of choosing a baked goody lingered. "I'll have that one please. Chocolate, is it?" I asked innocently, pointing to a delectable item on the middle shelf. "Chocolate coffee twist," she muttered in monotone indifference, as if that should be obvious by looking at the thing. My choice seemed sweet enough and a reasonable accompaniment to my latte, or so I thought. I didn't realize the error in my choice of dessert until that night, when midnight rolled around, and I was too wide-eyed to get to sleep. My heart was pounding, my legs were twitching, my mind was racing, my thoughts were flashing, and my *dormez-vous* had gone missing. I tried everything I could think of to conjure up the sandman. I reviewed the boring lecture notes from earlier in the day. I took a warm bath and did some deep-breathing exercises. I remembered a relaxation trick my dad taught me, using progressive muscle relaxation, starting with my toes and working upwards to my nose. I even attempted meditating on the colour purple while humming "om" in the lotus position, but to no avail. I was utterly and completely awake, and painfully aware of every creak in the hallway and every lump in the mattress. Why couldn't I have been this awake during the lecture series, when I could've put it to some practical use? I watched the digital radio-alarm clock scroll through every minute of every hour, one after the other, with limitless time to reprimand myself on my choice of afternoon treat. Chocolate coffee twist? Yes, and quite a twist indeed: it was laced with caffeine, which combined with the afternoon latte, spelled grand theft of my forty winks that night.

Disturbed sleep is all too common and estimated to regularly frustrate over three million Canadians. Those suffering from insomnia have the best of intentions; they spend enough time in bed, but lack the sleep to show for it. The causes of poor sleep-quality are many and varied and can include difficulty initiating sleep because of the sensation of creepy, crawly, restless legs, common to those with diabetes or kidney disease, to difficulty staying asleep, as experienced by those with sleep apnea who are forced awake by obstructed airflow. Evidence shows that those complaining of insomnia are at heightened risk for developing high blood pressure and cardiovascular disease. So it's important to let your family doctor know if you're having persistent difficulty with sleep. Therapies are available that can help to break a bad cycle and improve your sleep quality, not to mention your life quality and the health of your blood vessels.

On Call Again, Naturally

Being on call for the coronary care unit has given me an exquisite appreciation for the central role of sleep in maintaining our general health. When I first got my pager, I was in my third year of medical school. It was very cool then, and I was proud to strut down the hospital hallways with my white lab coat unbuttoned, showing off the pager strapped to my side. I felt very important, like a somebody at Speedy Muffler King, until the darn thing started going off. Then my sense of significance faded behind a growing gloom of imprisonment. My pager would beep all the beepin' time: mealtime, movie-time, playtime, Miller time, and especially during sleep time. On nights that I was on call, I would place my pager on the side table and, with the readout facing me, I would turn off the light, lie back onto my pillow, send a wee prayer heavenward requesting a quiet night, and wait. Wait for the worst. It's hard to settle with a time bomb next to you, and some nights I simply couldn't. Usually the ear-piercing squawk would jolt me out of whatever stage of sleep I managed to enter. Seldom would I get to do any REM of significance. The next day at work would be a blur of robotically going through the motions. This is the time medical mistakes are most easily made.

As it turns out, our brains are really only good for about sixteen hours without sleep. After this we begin to zone out and even micro-doze, with repeated brief lapses in alertness, explaining why my "snap-to-it-ness" in the wee hours of a call night often lacked the snap. Twenty hours without sleep produces a slowed reaction time, similar to that of an impaired driver, a particularly worrisome issue for those who share the roads with sleepy long-haul truckers. The American National Highway Traffic Safety Administration cites sleep deprivation as the cause for over 100,000 crashes, injuries, and fatalities each year.[5] In light of that incriminating bit of evidence, today's medical trainees are given taxi chits after completing their overnight shifts in the hospital, so they can get home safely and do no harm in the process. We need to add "don't drift off and drive" to our safety imperative of "don't drink and drive," to foster safer roads, not to mention sidewalks. Major disasters including Chernobyl may have been avoided if sleep had been given the priority it deserves.

The Ins and Outs of the Rhythm Method

Our sleep pattern is based on an internal biological clock known as the circadian rhythm. Derived from the Latin words *circa*, around, and *dian*, day, circadian refers to events or things that span a full day, like the wall of always-fresh Tim Hortons doughnuts behind the counter. The circadian rhythm is the twenty-four-hour cycle that governs many of our physiologic processes, including blood pressure, hormonal levels, digestive secretions, and our all-important sleep. Circadian rhythms are believed to have originated in the earliest cells, where cell division was timed to occur at night to protect the unravelled, fragile DNA from daylight's damaging ultraviolet rays. Our circadian rhythm is set by the environmental factors of light and temperature, as well as by internal factors, including release of the hormone melatonin.

Credit goes to a Greek geographer for being the first to document this circadian phenomenon. Androsthenes of Thasus served as an officer under the cruel rule of Alexander the Great, mapping the Persian Gulf. While Alexander was spreading his influence by sword and misery, his young captain was making observations regarding the flora and fauna of the coastline. For some reason, the Indian tamarind tree caught his eye, and he described how its leaves would move in position with the time of the day, something like modern-day, computer-controlled solar panels. Centuries later, the British would also take interest in this same tree, not so much for idle speculation about nature's rhythms, but for adding that quintessential zing to HP Worcestershire sauce.

Shift work plays havoc with our circadian rhythm, and numerous studies have awoken us to the many health issues at stake. Risks of peptic ulcer disease, Alzheimer's, diabetes, and heart disease are all increased in those who have to burn the midnight oil to make a living. Considering that 20 percent of the workforce in industrialized countries works shifts, sleep deprivation likely contributes substantially to the burden of chronic disease in our society. A study examining the effects of sleep deficit in emergency response helicopter pilots showed that incomplete recuperation time between work shifts led to accumulated sleep deprivation. They recommended that pilots take a mandatory ten-hour rest period per day, and encouraged unrestricted sleep opportunities on days off.[6] If such a rest and sleep regimen is good for operators of helicopters, it's probably good for operators of motor vehicles as well, you and me included.

While travelling across time zones is an obvious additional way our sleep rhythm can be disrupted, few realize that even the annual one-hour daylight-saving-time change can knock it about. A noticeable increase in traffic accidents has been documented following the spring-ahead change in clocks, as we lose an hour from our already limited night's sleep. What's more, in our money-doesn't-sleep society, with artificial lights blazing around the clock and grocery and department stores hoping for twenty-four-hour business, we are incessantly exposed to a chaos of time cues that easily upset our normal sleep pattern. In the beginning, God separated light from dark, but, thanks to Thomas Edison and the consumer machine, we've managed to put them back together again. By confusing the natural signals that foster healthy sleep patterns, we have created a grey haze of sleep disturbance, disrupting the natural circadian rhythms that were designed to protect us. To reduce the toll on our health in general and on our cardiovascular health in particular, we need to recover these rhythms.

Re-Establishing Night Rhythm

- Remove TV/computer distractions from bedroom
- Keep the bedroom dark while sleeping
- Keep room quiet to sleep
- Consider ear-plugs or white-noise machine
- Turn down the volume on the phone before bed to minimize possibility of being awoken

- Retire to bed and rise at the same time, weekend or not
- Go to sleep early enough that you don't need the alarm clock to awaken

Deprivation of the Nation

Regular Rip Van Winkles we're not. When it comes to restorative sleep, most Canadian adults are running on empty. National Sleep Foundation data recorded at the turn of the last century indicate that we sleep an average of two fewer hours per night than our forebears did.[7] Granted, insomnia is an important issue, but the sleep problems of the masses have less to do with sleep dysfunction and more to do with sleep starvation. Upwards of 70 percent of North American adults and 85 percent of adolescents don't get enough hours of sleep each night (although the teens can at least sleep till noon on Saturdays). Our sleep environments may have improved somewhat from the pre-Posturepedic mattress days, but if we're not clocking in the horizontal hours, then our creature comforts are of limited value. Moms universally recommend eight hours of sleep a night, and current data on optimal sleep duration still supports this time-honoured, wise council.

Self-induced sleep deprivation has become a societal norm to cope with the ever-increasing demands on our North American lifestyles (who listens to their mothers, anyhow?). It is ironic that we've never had more leisure time than in our present era, yet we've never taken less time to sleep. I used to try to purposely reduce my sleep requirements when I was at university, so I'd have more time to study (nerd alert!). My unfounded rationale was that if I limited my sleeping hours to the bare minimum, I would sleep more efficiently. Like the adage "absence makes the heart grow fonder," I reckoned that some sleep deprivation might discipline my body to better lap up the zzzs, and foster a deeper sleep the moment my head hit the pillow. At my most extreme, I trimmed my sleeping hours down to four hours a night, studying until two in the morning and rising at 6:00 a.m. with a "Good Morning, Vietnam!" alarm. And, yes, I slept soundly. But my experiment backfired: the quality of my study time deteriorated. I was spending more time staring blankly at my texts than learning the material, and, not surprisingly, I was dog-tired all day long.

The error of my sleep-depriving ways was clarified for me one evening while doing some last-minute studying before a final exam. It was an evening exam, which didn't start until 8:00 p.m., giving me ample time to review my notes before the library closed at 7:00 p.m., and get my thoughts together with a fresh-air walk before the test. As was my practice, I hid myself away in a quiet corner of the library so as not to be disturbed by those less studious. But it was almost too quiet. So, in the hushed silence of my warm study carrel, despite the impending test and hard chair, I fell sound asleep on my books. When I awoke and wiped the drool puddle off my text, I realized that I had two fairly urgent problems to solve. One, I had only ten minutes to get across campus for my exam. Two, I needed to get out of the library before I could solve problem number one. While I was dozing, dreaming about organic chemistry formulas, the library had closed for the night, and all doors were locked. I fumbled my way through the darkened stacks and saw the red exit light over the fire escape door. "My lucky way out," I figured. If I wasn't awake before I pushed on the door handle, I was alert and orientated when the shrill ring of the alarm blared over my head. Clutching my books, I dashed down the stairs and out of the building into the library courtyard, but as I started to make haste to the exam hall I noticed there were other people also rushing. At first, I figured they were fellow students like me, late for the exam, until the flashlights were shone in my face and I was asked to "freeze." I had some explaining to do to the campus police who stopped me. Fortunately, they seemed more amused than anything. I think I looked so tired that the officers believed my story and let me go on to my exam with the quip that I should "use the library during *waking* hours only."

Sleep deprivation is damaging to mind and body, and it's not just an issue for those with sleep apnea, chronic insomnia, or night-shift work schedules. Long-term lack of either sleep quality or quantity is damaging for all of us. While we may be able to readily recover from an isolated all-nighter in the office or from a transatlantic sleepless plane flight with a shower and a shot of caffeine, repeated sleep deprivation can produce profound and long-lasting injury. When we don't give our bodies the sleep they need, things go wrong. Studies performed on young, healthy volunteers have documented that sleep-deprived subjects had susceptibility to mood disorders, development of annoying fibromyalgia-like aches and pains, symptoms compatible with the chronic fatigue syndrome, and vascular-injuring problems of elevated blood pressure and impaired sugar metabolism.[8] Blood vessel function has also been studied in the sleep lab. When volunteers are sleep deprived, their blood vessels suffer. Using indirect measures of nitric oxide production, it has been shown that changes in sleep result in changes in levels of this vascular protector.[9] One of the key culprits that link poor sleep behaviour with the jeopardy of our vascular health is the stress hormone cortisol. Stay tuned …

"Family Pet Saves Seven"

I was very proud to bring a copy of the *Barrie Banner*, detailing the heroics of our dog, to my grade four show-and-tell, along with the melted lamp from our fire-destroyed rec room. When I recall our house fire, my mother's staccato imperatives still ring in my ears. "Out of bed boys! There's a fire! Quick now, to the car!" No questions asked. I leapt from my top bunk to the floor and could feel the heat of warmed boards under my feet. As I darted down the hallway to the front door and out, I could smell the smoke and hear the crackling flames. All five of us kids scrambled across the snow-drifted driveway in our pajamas to the station wagon, where we huddled for comfort and watched in disbelief. "We wouldn't have made it out if Carmen hadn't woken me up," my dad confessed with quavering voice, petting our dog's head repeatedly. The sirens intensified to an almost unbearable pitch. Within minutes our front yard could've been the set for Steve

McQueen's *Towering Inferno*, with firefighters, hoses, trucks, and a gathering crowd of neighbours. My hands were visibly shaking and my heart was beating into my ears. Although it was only 4:00 a.m., I was wide awake and ready to move a mountain, if need be.

The physiological phenomenon responsible for my instant wakefulness, racing heart, and muscular readiness is referred to as the "fight-or-flight" response. When under threat, our bodies can respond with increased speed and strength, enabling rapid action, like escaping a fire or leaping clear of a large, charging dog with big, white fangs. This response is possible due to the rush of stress hormones released into circulation, setting in motion all that is needed to flee up a tree or stand your ground and fight to the death (as a physician, I highly recommend the flee option, for longevity's sake). Adrenalin is responsible for the initial superman response, as we leap tall buildings and stop speeding bullets. Cortisol also helps with this initial response, but continues to lend assistance in the refueling after the action, in preparation for next time. Called the "general adaptation syndrome" by Canadian endocrinologist Dr. Hans Selye, this physiological response is clearly lifesaving and, together with the skills of berry-picking and eyelash-batting, is most likely responsible for the successful evolution of our species.

In the remote past, physical dangers were part of the everyday struggle. Putting meat on the table was no simple task, and limited-resource conflicts usually meant warring with other villages. In that barbaric context, the acute stress response had an immediate physical outlet, and if you survived by climbing a tree to safety or giving Goliath a death-blow between the eyeballs, then the stress ended. Once normalcy resumed, adrenalin levels diminished, heart rate and blood pressure normalized, and life carried on. But in today's world of computer crashes, traffic jams, managerial staff meetings, and teen body-piercing, the stress never goes away. Persistent release of stress hormones is itself stressful on our bodies, particularly on our sleep patterns and our blood vessels. The trick with stress hormones is achieving the right level: not too little, so you can still escape the big dog charging, and not too much that you damage your cardiovascular health.

The Bronzed Berliner

When I was in Berlin for my honeymoon, I made a point of visiting the City Hall where President Kennedy gave his legendary *"Ich bin ein Berliner"* address in 1963. Later that same day, my wife and I were invited to a pub by some locals, who wanted to hear *alles* about the Rocky Mountains. They treated us to schnapps and draft beer as we described the picturesque hiking trails around Banff. Enchanted by their hospitality, I spontaneously inserted JFK's famous remark as we were leaving to show my appreciation.

"Ich bin ein Berliner," I said.

"You're a what?" one asked.

"He said he's a doughnut," the other said, laughing.

I didn't get their joke and looked over at my blushing bride for translation. As I found out, Kennedy's famous line was grammatically incorrect: to say that you're a citizen of a city or country, you don't insert the *ein*. Apparently, I was describing myself as some type of sugary doughnut called a Berliner (very tasty, but heavy on the trans fatty acids). So I stuck with English for the remainder of our travels through *Deutschland*, to avoid getting lost in translation.

Such a minor linguistic gaffe didn't reduce my admiration of JFK in the least. He was clearly a remarkably gifted leader with ample charisma and vision and, what's more, he accomplished his landmark initiatives despite significant medical ailments. What you may not know about the late great thirty-fifth president was that he supposedly suffered from a condition known as Addison's disease. Patients with this rare endocrine disorder struggle with reduced production of the stress hormone cortisol. Known also as the "bronze disease," because of the darkening of the skin that can occur, Addison's disease was uniformly fatal before the discovery of synthetic steroids during the Great Depression of the 1930s. But even with regular steroid treatment, patients with Addison's are at risk when under stress, since they can't produce cortisol on demand to meet the needs of the body under strain, be it physical or emotional. As president during the tumultuous 1960s, with its counter-cultural revolution, civil-rights awakening, and anti-war movement, JFK was exposed to stress aplenty. It's reported that President Kennedy collapsed on a number of occasions from low blood pressure due to the lack of protective, stress-hormone response. Like others in Addisonian crisis he required emergency steroid injections to help him survive. Too little stress hormone renders us incapable of facing life's battles. Even giants like JFK needed cortisol to cope.

Cortisol's Cruel Cornucopia

Stress hormones wanted? Not by the majority of North Americans — the vast, stressed-out majority. When it comes to meeting the needs of our environmental stressors, from negotiating downtown traffic to completing the Christmas shopping list, we've got plenty of cortisol to go around. In fact, there is too much for the health of our blood vessel lining. What's more, smoking increases the stress hormone cortisol to 35 percent above the stressed average. And it's not that the levels of the stress hormone are so high; it's that the levels are too constant. Because we are always under the gun, cortisol production is always turned on, and our blood vessels don't get much of a break. In biological systems, there needs to be ebb and a flow. As it is written in the wise book of Ecclesiastes, "for everything there is a season … a time to tear, and a time to sew." We're just so darn busy tearing around, we rob our bodies the opportunity to sew. It's the constant presence of cortisol in our circulation that wears down the lining and increases the risk of vascular injury and disease.

Dr. Harvey Cushing was the first to recognize and describe patients who suffered from uncontrolled cortisol production. It was over eighty years ago, in the golden era of medicine, when doctors used to carefully examine patients, well before the likes of Dr. Gregory House and his indiscriminate use of full-body MRI scanning. Cushing's patients all shared an unusual "weeble" look, with large, wobbly torsos, and thin, stick-like appendages, barely strong enough to keep them from falling down. Today, the most common cause of Cushing's syndrome is the chronic medicinal use of steroids for treatment of, for example, connective tissue disorders. But back in the days when Shirley Temple danced with Fred Astaire, the most common source of excess cortisol was from tumour production.

Cortisol is a glucocorticoid hormone made in the cortex, or outer layer, of the adrenal glands, located above each kidney. Secretion of cortisol typically follows a circadian rhythm, with highest levels during the day, to help us deal with all the small stuff, and lowest levels at night, when we're supposed to be sound asleep in dreamland. The term glucocorticoid refers to its ability to increase the sugar, glucose, in our blood stream for immediate energy use. Cortisol is responsible for much of the energy transactions involved in the fight-or-flight response: first, in mobilizing energy so we can act quickly in a pinch and, second, after we've fought or fled, helping to store up energy for the next emergency response. Cortisol's energy-mobilizing work involves the breakdown of muscle fibres, which are energy-rich tissues. The downside of this catabolic activity over the long haul is that muscle mass gets reduced. This is why those with cortisol-secreting tumours have such weak and wasted appendages. The high levels of cortisol continuously eat away at the muscle tissue, faster than it can be replaced. But there's more bad news. Cortisol works to increase energy stores in the form of fat, in general, and belly fat, in particular, since this is the easiest for the body to get at for future energy draw. In addition to the Pillsbury Doughboy jelly-belly, cortisol-induced fat produces the characteristic round "moon face" and prominent "buffalo hump" fat pads in patients with this disorder. When fat is laid down in the abdomen, it's referred to as visceral fat, which unfortunately not only looks bad, but *is* bad. In excess, visceral fat increases heart disease risk more than any other type of fat.

Patients with Cushing's syndrome also complain of increased male-pattern facial hair; prominent purple stretch marks covering their fattened abdomen; thin, fragile skin that bruises easily; severe insomnia; as well as reduced libido (can't sleep and uninterested in using one of the best remedies). But of greater concern than even these significant symptoms and physical stigma, is that patients with Cushing's syndrome develop high blood pressure and blood sugars levels, and are at a markedly increased risk for developing vascular disease. Most heart attacks in the general population occur in the early morning hours when cortisol levels rise, supporting the contention that too much cortisol is stressful on the lining of our all-important blood vessels.

Although most people's cortisol levels aren't high enough to cause all the physical changes seen in patients with Cushing's syndrome, sleep deprivation, compounded with our daily grind, can favour high blood pressure and increased abdominal girth. Many weight experts currently believe that our societal obesity epidemic may be partly related to sleep-deprivation induced, elevated cortisol levels. And what's more, elevated cortisol can cause sleep disturbance in its own right, producing a vicious cycle of stress increase leading to cortisol increase/sleep decrease/stress increase/cortisol increase/ sleep decrease, and so on. In the whirl and spin of my emergency work schedule, I often found myself stuck in the throes of such a cycle. On my post-call nights in particular, despite being physically and mentally exhausted, I was often too tired to fall asleep because of the stimulating effects of stress-induced cortisol.

We may not be able to see all the effects of elevated cortisol, but they're ongoing, notwithstanding, and vascular disease is heading our way unless we can do something to reduce the cortisol levels. For patients with cortisol-secreting tumours, that something is surgical removal of the tumour — cut along the dotted line and we have a cure! But as for the cortisol excess driven by stress and sleeplessness, we aren't able to heal with surgical steel. For most of us with sleep issues, solutions to improving our slumber and reducing cortisol levels lie not in the realm of surgery or sleeping pills, but rather in a practical reshuffling of our priorities. For example, developing bedtime rituals that include twenty minutes of reading or listening to soft music, eating a bowl of cereal, retiring and rising at the same time (weekends included) will all go further to optimize our sleep patterns than will relying upon drugs and gimmicks.

Attack of the Killer "Z" Drugs

We are a drug-obsessed, pill-popping generation: a pill for everything and everything in a pill. If you've got a headache or a sore back, too many jitters or too little oomph, an unhealthy diet or an unwanted paunch, a receding hairline or a nervous poodle (I've never seen a calm poodle), there's a pill with a promise to make it all better. But by reducing the complexity of human beings to mechanistic receptor sites and metabolites, we come to the erroneous conclusion that every malady, from the life-threatening to the whimsical, can be rectified with an appropriate dose of some medical cocktail. Such is the case for sleep disturbance, where selling sleeping pills is a gargantuan business. People in the United States spend upwards of $3.5 billion annually on sleeping-pill prescriptions, keeping their doctors busy writing the over 48 million prescriptions per year. And thanks to our frenetic, high-stress work schedules and aggressive marketing to a sleep-deprived culture, prescription writing for sleeping medications is also gaining ground in Canada with every waking hour.

Sleeping pills aren't unique to our modern, fast times. In ancient Egypt, chamomile was a well-recognized herbal remedy for sleep disturbance, and was even given religious plant status, consecrated to the sun god. Today chamomile remains a popular remedy for ailments ranging from tummy upset and halitosis to skin sores and hemorrhoids, and has retained its legendary status as a sleep aid. My mother-in-law loves to bring out the chamomile tea when we visit. She regularly replenishes her supplies with each trip to Germany, where I understand the Germans revere it like Asians do ginseng.

The ancient Greeks also had their sleep remedies. If counting Greek gods jumping over Mount Olympus failed to bring on slumber, they turned to the soporific properties of valerian root. The great physician Galen frequently prescribed the dried valerian root (which remains the active ingredient in today's over-the-counter Nytol preparation), for treating insomnia. In medieval times, valerian root made the top ten list of essential herbs in the alchemist's grotto.

Legend has it that valerian root was up the sleeve of the Pied Piper of Hamelin. When his flute-playing wasn't cutting it with the rodents, the rat-catcher used the fragrance of valerian root to help attract the rats to the river for their drowning. Unfortunately, the effectiveness of his herbal remedy didn't win him many brownie points with the townspeople, who refused to pay his exterminator fee, and forced his hand to abscond with their next of kin.

In addition to the numerous herbal products that are available today for sleep induction (row upon row in your local health food store), there is a seemingly endless array of other products for conjuring up the god of slumber. They include powdered milk baths, pillow and room fragrant sprays, sleepy-time beverages such as S'nores chocolate milk and Crème de la REM with melatonin and lactium, and rosemary and peppermint aromatic oils. But if these aren't strong enough to knock you into dreamland, there are numerous powerful modern-day prescription sedatives which have undergone considerable refinement over the years, as the pharmaceutical industry has been searching for the most effective and least toxic magic bullet for sleep induction. The barbiturates were the first to be developed. Their name is derived from St. Barbara, the patron saint of artillerymen — an unusual choice for a sedating drug, unless you're the type who sleeps with a pistol under the pillow. An early form called barbital was too strong for human consumption, but found a niche market in the canine community, used by veterinarians to put down dogs. In 1912, the more refined phenobarbital was introduced as a sedative, and remained popular into the 1950s, despite its many side effects, including dizziness, depression, daytime fatigue, and decreased libido. In the 1940s the rival drug chloral hydrate gained popularity, due in part to the brilliant performance of Humphrey Bogart in the film noir classic *The Maltese Falcon*. He played the private eye Sam Spade and used the drug to disarm his suspects. The drug was referred to as a Mickey Finn, named after the sneaky bartender who would slip it into the drinks of the unsuspecting bad guys. But with growing bad press about side effects of and dependence on these drugs, intensified by Marilyn Monroe's overdose, interest shifted to the more sophisticated sedative class benzodiazepine, of which valium (diazepam), ativan (lorazepam), and estazolam (found in Sleepees) are examples. In the 1970s these were the sedatives of choice, filling the medicine cabinets of neurotic North Americans. More recently, the blockbuster Z drugs have swept the sleep-crazed market as the newest generation in sleeping pills, including zolipdem (Ambien) and eszopiclone (Lunesta), promising an even better night's sleep.

Problems with all these sleep aids are many and include the masking of more serious problems, like depression, anxiety disorders, and eating disorders.[10] As well, powerful sedatives like these tend to depress breathing. People with sleep apnea are at particular risk since sedatives can make the no breathing sleep apnea pauses longer, even to the point of no return. In careless combination with alcohol, sedatives can be deadly. The Heaven's Gate Cult took advantage of this bit of physiology when they asphyxiated themselves to board the near approaching Hale-Bopp comet. There are over 1,000 deaths annually in North America from sedative-induced asphyxiation. Hank Williams cut his honky-tonk blues career short this way and Jimi Hendrix probably did the same.

Even when taken as directed, sleeping pills don't stop working just because the sun rises. They continue to do the same thing in the day as they do at night — namely, create a fog. Regular use of sleeping pills reduces memory, judgment, and energy levels. And the frustrating thing is that despite the expense and side effects, sleeping pills don't improve the brain's sleep-cycle wave pattern. As a result, the pill approach doesn't induce sleep that is refreshing or address the underlying reasons for the sleeping difficulty, such as restless leg syndrome or sleep apnea.

Last and very important, sleeping pills are habit-forming drugs. You're already trying to kick the tobacco addiction with its nicotine stranglehold on your brain. Why get hooked on some sleep aid that's also difficult to quit? As my children remind me when they drift off into slumber, sleeping is a natural state, like happiness. And like happiness, we shouldn't have to force it to happen with drugs. The vast majority of us with sleeping difficulties are better off without the use of sedatives. If you take sleeping pills regularly, you may be dependent currently, and would be wise to quit as soon as possible. Be aware, however, that abrupt discontinuation of sleeping pills can produce trouble. In particular, stopping the benzodiazepine class cold turkey can cause withdrawal symptoms similar to what alcoholics experience in the dry tank, including anxiety, dizziness, depression, night sweats, palpitations, and rebound insomnia.[11] Although these symptoms are more likely if you've been on high doses for long periods of time, the symptoms have also been noted to occur in patients receiving recommended doses for short-term therapy. Tapering the dose can help in the process of weaning off sleeping-pill dependence. As well, mild sedatives, like Nytol's valerian root, are useful as a transition medication when you're coming clean.

If you're having difficultly falling asleep, helpful sleep hygiene suggestions abound, like drawing a warm bath or reading quietly before retiring. But an essential place to start is to reduce the stimulants on our minds and bodies. This includes cutting out the bedtime smoking, because nicotine is a stimulant.

Things to Avoid for a Sound Sleep

- nicotine
- coffee, black tea, cola (caffeine)
- dark chocolate (caffeine)
- guarana (caffeine)
- ephedra (ma huang), a stimulant
- cold decongestants containing Synephrine
- bitter orange (citrus aurantium) contains Synephrine
- heavy meals before bed
- heavy alcohol consumption before bed
- exercising within four hours of sleeping
- watching TV, news, loud music before bed

Putting the "Good" Back into "Night"

"As a smoker, you're sort of between a rock and a hard place when it comes to sleep," I levelled with Peter. "The problem is, nicotine tends to disrupt deep sleep, whether it comes from cigarettes or from nicotine replacement therapy, like the patch. For that matter, so can bupropion (Zyban) and even cold turkey nicotine withdrawal, possibly explaining some people's smoking cessation failures."

"So maybe I should just keep smoking and take my chances with the cigarette nicotine," Peter said playfully.

"I don't think so," I countered. "What it really means is that optimal sleep patterns are important to have in place while you begin the process of quitting, since nicotine withdrawal may add further challenge. Despite the transient effect on sleeping, quitting is by far the healthiest option. Besides, the withdrawal part is only temporary, lasting at the most three to four weeks. So I would strongly encourage you to keep the idea of quitting on the front burners. And don't forget, after merely eight hours of slumber, your body is nicotine-free and already beginning to recover from the previous day's cigarette damage."

"So what about improving my sleep?" Peter asked. "Any other suggestions, other than avoiding nicotine before bed?"

"Well, to begin with," I offered, "you might want to limit your afternoon snoozing. Albert Einstein supposedly took catnaps, and he was a pretty smart guy. But daytime napping tends to disrupt the circadian sleep rhythm and diminish sleep quality. It's probably better just to push through the day and retire all the earlier if you're really bushed. You know, Benjamin Franklin's adage 'early to bed and early to rise.'"

"What about the sleep apnea possibility that you mentioned earlier?" his attentive daughter asked me. "Does Dad need some special tests or treatment for that?"

"Your symptoms of daytime fatigue and nighttime, sawmill snoring certainly could be related to a sleep disorder like sleep apnea," I told Peter, "but I'm no expert in the field. Let's have you fill out this

You Snooze or You Lose

Epworth Sleepiness Questionnaire." I handed the questionnaire to him for review.[12] "For the situations listed, rate your likelihood of falling asleep, between zero, for 'never,' and three, for 'definite,' and go over the results with your family doctor. The questionnaire helps to give us an idea if you're getting enough sleep or not, and if something more serious is going on. Eight hours isn't enough for some, while others thrive on less sleep. If your score cracks 10, then further investigations may be warranted to look into the sleep apnea concern."

Epworth Sleepiness Questionnaire

Situation	Chance of Sleeping
1. Sitting and reading	
2. Watching TV	
3. Sitting inactive in a public place	
4. Being a passenger in a vehicle for over an hour	
5. Lying down in the afternoon	
6. Sitting and talking with someone	
7. Sitting quietly after lunch (no alcohol)	
8. Stopped for a few minutes in traffic while driving	

Score: 0 = never; 1 = slight; 2 = moderate; 3 = definite

Total score	Interpretation
1–6	Rested
7–8	Borderline
9–10	Sleep-Deprived
>10	At Risk for Sleep Disorder

Source: Epworth Sleepiness Score courtesy of M.W. Johns, "A New Method for Measuring Daytime Sleepiness: The Epworth Sleepiness Scale." *Sleep* 14(6) (1991): 540–45.

TOOTH FAIRY CONFIDENTIAL

No Lost Cause

As soon as I stepped into the consultation room, I could immediately sense the tension. Peter was standing next to the exam table, arms folded and eyes evading mine. "Don't tell me, you're still smoking and figure I'm gonna tear you to bits?" I asked as I sat down beside him.

"Well, yeah," Peter said, wincing. "But I figured, what's the point of even trying to quit. I mean, my dad died at age sixty-two, Mom at sixty-six, and now my younger brother. My days are numbered, so why should I bother quitting? And besides, we've all gotta go sometime. If it's because of smoking or being hit by a bus, what's the difference anyways?"

I grinned. "The cleanup crew might have an opinion on that. But fortunately for us, we're not deciding between modes of death. It's life that holds my interest. I'm committed to life in general and yours in particular. You're not a lost cause," I emphasized. "You've got a family, and you're relatively young and active, with lots on the go. Your story doesn't have to end suddenly. It's too premature to be talking obituary. There's still much that you can do to help reduce your risk of heart disease. Let's take another look at the PLAC diagram, for example."

I pulled out my cross-sectional diagram of the blood vessel again, showing the four regions where disease strikes. Pointing to number one, I said, "We've hit the platelets already with your daily Aspirin and omega-3 capsules. As for protecting the vascular lining, we discussed the importance of sleep hygiene, and you're on the blood pressure pill that I prescribed, right?"

Peter nodded a "yes," with a facial expression that said "reluctantly."

"According to today's blood pressure reading of 132/82 mmHg, it looks like you've got reasonable control happening on that front," I said, putting a check mark beside number two. "And there are more ways to reduce your chances of having a heart attack or stroke. That is, *in addition* to quitting smoking cigarettes, there are some other strategies to help reduce your risk."

"Who says I'm quitting?" Peter asked in a tone reminiscent of Joe Pesci in *Goodfellas*.

I smiled. "I'm a wishful thinker. And to help see my wish come true — namely you at a lower risk for having a vascular calamity — we should move on to number three on the PLAC diagram," I suggested as I circled Active Inflammation (see the little x marks on the figure). Heart disease is an inflammatory disorder. To protect ourselves from heart attack and stroke, we need to reduce the amount of inflammation coming at our blood vessels.

Red-Hot and Swollen

My first recollection of the inflammatory response was when I was playing scooter tag with some friends and wiped out on the gravel road in front of our house. As my mom consoled me and swabbed the scrape on my leg with peroxide solution, she explained

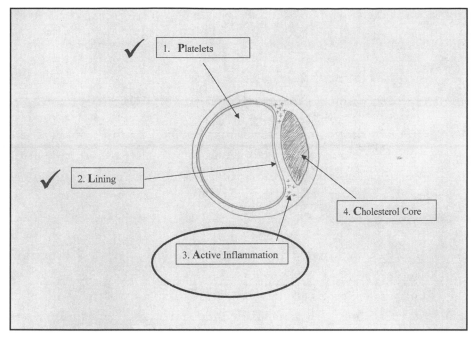

Figure 5.1: Active inflammation.

that my "owie was red and painful because the 'good guy' blood cells were fighting off the 'bad guy' bacteria to make it all better again." Although the cellular response to injury is more complex than merely a fight between good and bad forces, it's an explanation that I've since used with my own kids after their tumbles.

Inflammation is the body's programmed response to injury, whether from physical trauma, like my scooter accident, or from infection, burn, toxin exposure, frostbite, or some other mischief. The physical features of inflammation, including redness, swelling, heat, and pain, have been well described since ancient Greek times when Celsus noted them in 30 B.C.E. — possibly also following a scooter incident. The inflammatory response is under the control and direction of our immune system. It is designed to protect our bodies from disease, namely infections and cancer. The efficiency of our immune system in undertaking this vitally important task is enough to make the most advanced twenty-first-century security forces blush. Our circulatory system is under constant surveillance by patrolling white blood cells that meticulously inspect every nook and cranny of our body for signs of tumour cells or pathogens, such as bacteria, viruses, or parasites. Day and night these immune cells keep vigil, combing the surface of each of our healthy cells and tissues, looking for evidence of foreign material that might signify a breach of security. If bacteria or viruses are detected, the body responds with prompt and extreme prejudice. Like disturbing an ant nest, the activated white cells sound the red alert to rally an instant and vast cellular army to the rescue. Blood vessels dilate to speed the arrival of fighter cells to the area under attack, causing the area to swell and become reddened and warm to the touch.

Harry Kleiner's 1966 sci-fi thriller *The Fantastic Voyage* dramatically illustrated this immune cell triggering process. Predating nanotechnology, the film portrayed a miniaturized Raquel Welch and her medical colleagues travelling in a cheesy spaceship through the vasculature of a critically injured diplomat. Their mission was to save his life from the inside. When the ship broke down, the patrolling white cells were alerted. Depicted as monstrous blobs, the immune cells attacked the crew, ingesting everything foreign in their path. Although a bit dated by *Star Wars* standards, the movie was a landmark in its day, taking the viewer down to the cellular level and into the realm of inflammatory battle.

Much Ado About Nothing

Unless we live out our lives isolated from contact with the outside world like the unfortunate Ted DeVita or David Vetter did in plastic bubbles, we need a well-functioning immune system to keep infections at bay. While the immune system's acute inflammatory response is critical for our health and survival, it can be the source of significant problems if it gets triggered inappropriately. Say hello to allergy. The prime example of abnormal activation of our immune system is the allergic reaction. This irritating phenomenon occurs because some people's immune systems are wired far too tightly and they overreact to otherwise harmless environmental stimuli, or allergens. The triggered inflammatory response is usually quite sudden, with symptoms that can take the form of annoying hives, or the itchy eyes and runny nose of hay fever, to more serious symptoms of asthmatic shortness of breath and wheezing, and the potentially fatal vascular collapse and respiratory failure of anaphylactic shock. Short of trying to limit exposure to known allergens, the mainstay of medical management for allergies is to turn off or at least dampen this unnecessary inflammatory reaction.

I learned about the anguish of inappropriate inflammation the winter I discovered I had a tape allergy. Like most great discoveries, it was rather serendipitous. My parents' second-storey bathroom window wouldn't shut properly. As a wannabe handyman, I climbed up onto the snowy rooftop to try my hand at repair. Ignorant of the maxim that "for every action there is an equal and opposite reaction," I pounded my fist on the frame to get it closed. But as it turned out, the force I used to hit the window frame was equal, but in the opposite direction to, the force that caused my feet to slip out from under me. I made a mental note to review that chapter in my physics text as I fell off the roof, plummeting into the drifts below and twisting my ankle in the process. After X-rays confirmed that it wasn't broken, the medic taped my ankle for support, from my toes to just below the knee. The sprain healed uneventfully over the next few days, but when I peeled off the tape I noticed that my skin was a bright red (not to mention warm and very itchy) underneath. The next day my leg was even warmer, itchier, more reddened, and quite swollen — so swollen, in fact, that I couldn't even fit on my shoe. I had to do the one-foot-in-a-baggie routine for the better part of a week, limping around like a plastic-wrapped pirate. It was the chemicals in the tape adhesive that set off an inflammatory response with my skin. The tape-allergy injury was far more impressive than the trauma I suffered from my rooftop drop. If I had simply iced my sprained ankle and skipped the medic's taping effort, I would've been dancing the light fantastic a lot sooner than I could have with my inflamed peg leg.

The phenomenon of allergy highlights two important lessons about our body's inflammatory response. Firstly, the body doesn't always know what's good for it. Even seemingly harmless stimuli, such as mould blowing in the spring wind, cat saliva from brushing up against Mr. Bigglesworth, or the minutest amount of stinger venom from an angered bumblebee, can set off the inflammatory response. In such cases, the inflammatory triggering can be inappropriate and not at all in our best interests. Second, once turned on, the response can be more damaging on the body than the stimulus would have been if it had simply been ignored by our immune system. Although the original design of the inflammatory response is to help in the cleanup and repair following an injury, its effects can be damaging, despite the best of intentions.

In recent years, researchers have also noted that inflammation was occurring within the walls of our blood vessels. Although it's not an allergic response, it is, nonetheless, a very poor choice of locale for such activity. It's no fault of the white blood cells; they're just following orders. The problem is that there are too many orders. In our sedentary society there are numerous inflammatory triggers that continually bombard our immune system and turn on white cell activity. And the party place is the wall of our blood vessels. As it turns out, vascular inflammation disrupts the normal functioning of the blood vessels and accelerates vascular plaque formation. It is currently understood that this inflammation contributes significantly to the development of atherosclerosis and, ultimately, to the vast number of heart attacks and strokes in our fair land.[1]

Whoa There! I Say, Whoa!

It was a sweltering hot day on the family farm, and my grandpa was giving Dad a hard time, since he was doing all the hard work repairing some fencing, while his son was merely sitting on the tractor, tilling the soil.

"Not fair that old men have to do all the back-breaking labour and lazy boys sit and putter," Gramps tauntingly said.

"Well, I don't mind trading jobs," my dad replied, catching the old man off guard, since they both knew full well he couldn't drive the tractor.

"You don't think I can do it?" Grandpa said defensively.

"Why, sure you can do it, Pop," reassured Dad. "There's nothing to it. See, here's the throttle and brake, and you steer with the wheel, like this."

So Grandpa, raised on a horse and buggy, hesitantly climbed up onto the tractor to try his hand at puttering. And as he slowly rolled his way along the row, Dad picked up the next fence boards for hammering. The long, straight row was no difficulty for the novice driver, but when Grandpa came to the corner, he failed to compensate for the tractor's generous turning radius. He turned the wheel too late to affect the tractor's forward momentum and he began to skid sideways. Flustered, Grandpa instinctively pulled up on the steering wheel and yelled, "Whoa! I say, whoa!" as the tractor turned right into the newly repaired fence. "Put on the brake!" Dad yelled to his father, but to no avail. The tractor tore down fifty metres of fence before Dad could jump on and apply the brakes. Grandpa never complained about his appointed tasks again.

Certain diseases called autoimmune disorders act like the farming tractor tearing down the farmer's good fencing. In such cases, the body loses its ability to recognize itself as *itself*. As a result, an inflammatory response gets triggered and is directed towards the person's own cells and tissues. As if in a cellular civil war, the immune machinery turns against its own body. By contrast to allergic reactions, these self-directed attacks aren't usually as sudden and explosive, but more often cause their damage in a slow and persistent fashion. With no brakes applied, this chronic inflammation can produce severe injury to the body over time. Connective tissue diseases such as rheumatoid arthritis and lupus (systemic lupus erythematosus or SLE) are examples of autoimmune diseases that can cause disabling joint destruction and organ damage by attacking the self as if it were a foreign intruder. This inflammatory havoc damages the heart and blood vessels. It's been shown that patients with rheumatoid arthritis and lupus are more prone to developing atherosclerotic vascular injury, due to the chronic inflammation in their bodies.

Inflammation-O-Meter

When the inflammatory response gets fired up, the liver snaps into action to help the white blood cells eradicate the enemy. The liver produces an array of proteins called acute phase reactants that bind onto invading bacteria and viruses, providing the white blood cells something to grab onto. These are also referred to as complement proteins and can be routinely measured in the blood. The best known complement protein is the C-reactive protein, or CRP. It was first identified during the Great Depression, shortly after Sir Alexander Fleming discovered penicillin. Overshadowed by the success of the life-saving antibiotic, CRP didn't get much attention at the time. However, in more recent times, it has earned its place in the laboratory armamentarium as a useful marker for inflammation. Levels of CRP rise dramatically when there is an infection, especially a bacterial infection, and fall with resolution of the illness. As a result, CRP levels are commonly measured to help chart a patient's progress with medical therapy.

With current technological advances, we can now measure even the tiniest elevations in CRP levels. It has recently been appreciated that these very low levels of CRP are not normal and represent low-grade, grumbling inflammation in the body. Cardiologists started to take note when it was shown that these low levels of CRP were associated with an increased risk of heart disease.[2] This relationship has helped foster the growing acceptance that vascular disease is due at least in part to the damaging effects of the inflammatory process. This realization has refined our understanding of how and why heart attacks happen. Current study is underway to determine the potential sources of smouldering inflammation that can lead to vascular damage, so that they can be effectively doused.[3]

One newly rediscovered source of inflammation is our mouths, especially mouths that have been neglected. Dental plaque and diseased gums not only give bacteria a safe haven to damage our teeth, but also an opportunity to raise the bar of inflammation throughout our bodies. It has been shown that bacterial toxins from our mouths can gain access to our bloodstream through diseased gums.[4] Our immune system reacts to these toxins by increasing the number of patrolling white blood cells that circulate through our bodies and inadvertently bring harm to our blood vessels. People with gum disease not only have higher levels of inflammation in their mouths, but have more inflammation in their bloodstream, accompanied by elevated CRP levels. But there is good news as well. It has been clearly demonstrated that when people with inflamed gums and high CRP levels undergo dental cleaning, the inflammation subsides, and their CRP levels return to normal.[5] So it's not just the dentists who need to say "you really should be brushing more thoroughly and flossing every day." Poor dental hygiene increases inflammation in our blood vessels and is a significant health liability.

The Bite Is Worse Than the Bark

"It's better to be bitten by a dog than by a person, you know," the owner of the chihuahua said as she gained control of her miniature monster. The dog's attack was partly my fault. I hadn't realized that the front door of the house was ajar when I opened the outside screen door to deliver the weekly newspaper. And before I could defend myself, little Tinkles was all over my ankle, gnawing at it like a rawhide bone covered in bacon drippings. "A dog's mouth doesn't have nearly the number of bacteria that a human mouth has," she went on to say as I held my bleeding ankle. Her attempts at comforting reassurance didn't ease the pain much. In fact, pondering the number of bacteria in a dog's mouth wasn't even remotely on my radar screen. The only incoming message that my brain was receiving was "ow, my ankle hurts." But I did make a mental note to keep a safe distance from potential biters, man and beast alike. And from then on, I delivered my newspapers with heightened caution. I kept a tightly rolled-up newspaper in my delivery bag, ready to draw at any moment with the words of Robert Baden-Powell ringing in my ears, "Be prepared!"

The chihuahua owner was right. Our mouths contain a vast number of bacteria, with representatives from over five hundred different species. Like a microscopic United Nations Assembly, our mouth is a busy place, with each group of bacteria continually vying for a foothold on our pearly whites and gums. And even the most obsessive Listerine gargler has a mouthful. Mouthwash may knock down the bacterial count temporarily, but no matter what we do, we just can't sterilize our mouths. Like the proverbial cat, bacteria keep coming back. With a nearly constant temperature of 37 degrees Celsius and a guaranteed 100 percent humidity, our mouths are a warm and wet jungle, the perfect paradise for germs to be fruitful and multiply. Rabbits have nothing on oral bacteria. With a generation time of fifteen to twenty minutes, it doesn't take long for bacterial numbers to be in bust mode again shortly after a swish of mouthwash.

Some dentists recommend chewing gum to increase saliva production (sugarless gum that is). The average three pints of saliva we make in our mouths daily can help wash bacteria into our throats and down to an acidic grave in our stomachs. As well, our saliva contains antibodies and enzymes that inhibit growth of certain fungi and bacteria. But that being said, there are other microbes that capitalize on substances in our saliva to actually boost their numbers.[6] Although secreted sterile from our glands, by the time our saliva settles on our molars, every millilitre is home to tens of millions of bacteria. All told, it is estimated that we each have more bacteria in our mouths than there are people on the planet. The greatest number of bacteria occurs in the morning before brushing, with nearly half of them attached to our tongue. This likely explains why only our pet dog wants to kiss me when I first get up in the morning.

Heart Sick

During my early medical training, I was introduced to the potential dangers of mouth bacteria. It was a challenging case of fever of unknown origin. My senior resident asked me to help admit a patient with a fever to the hospital. He said he needed more time to carefully examine some nubile cheerleader's sprained ankle, so he gave me the chart for the patient who was thermally hot. The patient with the fever was a hefty, middle-aged man who had pungent body odor and teeth like those of Austin Powers, minus the smile. His story was vague in description: fatigue, fever, chills, all increasing over the past number of weeks. His large, sweaty body was a challenge to examine (give me a straightforward ankle assessment, any day), but I did my best to consider the diagnostic possibilities for his fever, and sent off blood samples and a throat swab for lab assessment.

Our initial clinical assessment failed to offer a diagnosis as to the cause of his fever. He was surely infected by some bug, somewhere, but we couldn't determine the cause or origin of his infection. In cases like these, medics often resort to using empiric antibiotics. In my case, as a medical student, *empiric* meant that I "got-no-clue-what-I'm-treating." When applied to antibiotics, empiric usually involves using a combination of drugs to cover a broad range of infectious possibilities. Lo and behold, the patient improved on my drug regimen. His fever broke, and within a couple of days he started to eat and move about.

A few days later the patient's lab results came in and confirmed that he was, indeed, infected. He had a bacterial infection in his bloodstream, causing his initial fever. The bacteria responsible were identified as one of the *Streptococcus mutans* group. These round, microscopic creatures live by the motto "strength in numbers" and attach to each other in long chains. They are found in high numbers in our mouths and are responsible for the majority of our dental caries. Knowing the culprit bacteria, we were able to fine-tune the antibiotic medicines to finish off the remaining bacteria. Caesar's terse remark "I came, I saw, I conquered" came to mind. "My job is done!" I proudly thought. But my smugness didn't last long; the patient's clinical improvement was short-lived.

"He's spiking a temperature again," the charge nurse nagged, "and he doesn't want to eat his dinner."

Glancing at the meal tray of shepherd's pie that looked more like a dog's breakfast, I replied, "Well, at least he hasn't lost his mind."

But she was right. Despite appropriate doses of intravenous antibiotics targeted at the culprit bacteria, his condition was worsening. His fever came back, and, to make matters worse, he was now complaining of being short of breath. Even just sitting in his chair he was huffing and puffing as if he had just run a race. An old medical maxim came to mind: "When in doubt, examine the patient." So we did look him over again, and on this assessment we discovered that his heart was failing and his lungs were full of fluid, explaining his breathlessness. Ultrasound imaging of his heart gave us the answer to why he was deteriorating. On one of his heart valves there was a large clump of material that looked like laundry fluttering on a clothesline.

"What on earth is that?" I asked my senior resident.

"He's got endocarditis," he replied. "His heart valve is infected, and that clump is called a vegetation, full of bacteria. He's going to need surgery to clear this infection," he added in a sombre tone.

"But how did it get there?" I innocently inquired.

"Probably his teeth," my resident replied. "Did you see his mouth? Probably hasn't seen a toothbrush since Ed Sullivan," he added with a shiver.

An X-ray of his mouth confirmed three abscesses. Puzzle solved: his infected mouth allowed bacteria to get into his bloodstream and set up home on his heart valve, which finally gave out, explaining his worsening symptoms.

Before the advent of antibiotics in the 1940s, endocarditis was uniformly fatal. In the days when Henry Ford was painting his cars black, such patients were admitted for palliative care, as terminal cancer patients are today. Even in our modern era of prompt diagnosis, state-of-the-art medical imaging, powerful therapies, and routine open-heart surgery, infective endocarditis continues to carry substantial risk of illness and even death.[7] Our approach has been to prevent heart-valve infection by having those people with known heart valve abnormalities take an antibiotic every time they have a dental procedure. The rationale was based on the fact that bacteria can gain access to our bloodstream during dental manipulation and that abnormally functioning heart valves are more likely to get infected if they do. But these efforts haven't done much to avert infection. As it turns out, bacteria can get from our mouths to our blood vessels, even when the dentist isn't drilling. Oral bacteria can make the migration while you're eating a meal, chewing gum, or clenching your teeth over a traffic jam. The surest way to a man's heart may be through his stomach, but bacteria get there by way of diseased gums. So rather than prescribing antibiotics for prevention, we're supporting our dental colleagues and raising the banner for improved dental hygiene for all.[8] If we reduce the number of bacteria in our mouths and improve the health of our gums, the risk of bacteria gaining entrance into our bloodstream and causing infection drops significantly.

We sent our patient for open-heart surgery to remove the heart valve vegetation. At the time of surgery, the valve was caked in pus and completely destroyed. The surgical team had to replace the infected valve with an artificial one. Analysis of the infected valve showed *Streptococcus mutans* bacteria, just like that we had found in his blood and knew was heavily represented in his foul mouth. Despite a rocky hospital course and eight more weeks of hospital food, he recovered to tell the tale. As for me and my bruised medical ego, I gained a whole, new appreciation for the importance of proper dental hygiene.

Plaque Calls to Plaque

Even if bacteria don't gain entrance into our bloodstream directly to cause heart valve infection, like the one my patient managed to contract, oral bacteria can also have indirect, damaging effects on other parts of our cardiovascular system. Poor dental hygiene can allow bacteria to flourish in our mouths and allow their toxic by-products to accumulate. These toxins can spill into our bloodstream across damaged gums, turn on our inflammatory machinery, and do a number on our blood vessels.

The bacterial bastion from which the mouth microbes launch their attack is dental plaque: very different in composition from the plaque in our blood vessels, but, as it turns out, also at fault in causing heart disease. Bacteria get their start by first adhering to the neck of our teeth, forming a white biofilm.[9] You can see this on your dental floss if your technique is good, especially if you let a few days go by without flossing. If you don't floss, the biofilm develops into mushroom-like tunnels from the breakdown of sugar.[10] Firmly attached to our teeth, the bacteria happily live out their lives, eat our sweets, multiply faster than rabbits, and hide from superficial attempts at brushing. If left unperturbed, these purchases become hard, resembling barnacles on the underside of a boat. As part of our dental landscape, they then attract more bacterial colonies, complete with residential subdivisions, school, and community hall. They convert dietary sugar into acidic products that not only cause cavities, bad breath, and discolouration of the teeth, but also irritate our gums. If you examine your mouth in the mirror, the gum tissue next to your teeth should be light pink, blanching with pressure from your finger. With gum inflammation, this interface becomes reddened and prone to bleeding. This is referred to as periodontitis, and as it progresses in severity, the bacteria invade deeper into the tissue layers surrounding the teeth. Eventually, the bacteria, or at least their toxic waste products, find their way into our circulatory system, turn on the white blood cell inflammatory machinery, and raise havoc with our blood vessel linings. Since dental plaque can then lead to vascular plaque, our heart health focus needs to include improvements in dental care. If we want to reduce the risk of heart attack and stroke, we'll need to stop oral bacteria from completing their mission: "Today the mouth, tomorrow the world!"

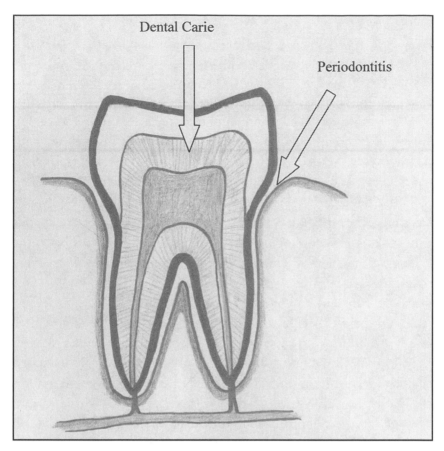

Figure 5.2: Dental access sites for bacteria.

Smiles Under Attack

In the First World War, the soldiers on the front lines came down with terrible oral infections. Under the constant emotional stress of battle and sleep deprivation, and in the midst of crowded unsanitary conditions, with only bad food and cigarettes to provide any diversion, they were perfect targets for enemies of the microscopic variety. One common contagion that they endured amid gunfire and black flak was a severe gum infection called ulcerative gingivitis. Still referred to today as trench mouth, this painful condition is marked by grey ulcerations around the gums that make talking and swallowing difficult. Trench mouth caused deterioration of gums and supporting bone tissue and, without treatment, resulted in the loss of teeth. But you don't need to contract trench mouth to lose teeth. Smoking increases the risk of tooth loss.

Oral health problems and smoking are like peanut butter and jelly — they commonly go together. And it's not just yellow teeth or bad breath. Smoking increases the risk of gum disease, facial pain, tooth decay, and dental loss. Over half of gum infections are related to either damage from current smoking or damage from previous smoking exposure. This explains why those who smoke are at four times the risk for developing periodontitis.[11] Before fumes reach the lungs to create havoc there, smoke injures our oral tissues by a variety of means. Firstly, there's the heat from the cigarette smoke. Our gums are temperature sensitive and designed for 37 degrees Celsius. Although hardy enough to handle occasional sips of tea and coffee or a hot toddy, the repeated inhaling of a smouldering cigarette goes beyond the normal health boundaries for our gums. The increased temperature in the mouth from smoking cigarettes directly injures the gums, especially around the base of the teeth. This constant damage renders the protecting gum tissue less able to stay attached to the teeth. And the more our teeth are exposed to the damaging effects of bacteria and their acidic toxins, the more vulnerable they become to decay. Secondly, there's the gas exposure. With each drag, the mouth is filled with a high concentration of burnt toxic fumes. The oral tissues are choked by carbon monoxide and starved of oxygen. The reduced oxygen delivery to the gums weakens the tissue's defence mechanisms, giving further advantage to resident bacteria. Thirdly, there's the issue of nicotine exposure on the gums. This chief addictive ingredient in cigarettes impairs the natural repair system in our mouths. Both production of collagen, a central repair protein, and formation of new bone are reduced in the mouths of those who smoke. Because of impaired healing capacity, microscopic wear-and-tear injuries in the mouth are less apt to mend properly and more likely to serve as an entrance for bacteria and their toxins. As a result, smoking gives oral bacteria an upper hand in causing dental damage and a solid foothold for invading our bloodstream.[12]

But it's not all doom and gloom for the mouth of a resolute smoker. Even though smoking cessation is the single most effective means of improving dental hygiene, some earnest attention to regular preventative care can take you a long way in the right direction. While experiments have confirmed that smokers with gum disease have impaired blood vessel functioning and are at higher risk for heart attack and stroke, it has also been shown that those same blood vessels can enjoy improved function after some solid dental hygiene practices — even if you continue to smoke.[13] So why neglect your mouth? It's taking the first hit with every drag, so it deserves a little Rodney Dangerfield respect. Although it's never too late to quit smoking, the benefits of dental care wane sharply after one's teeth fall out. So don't wait to put some muscle where your mouth is. Improving oral health needs to be a health priority for all who smoke and for all who successfully quit.

The Dental Trinity

Every time I darken the door of my dentist, I'm reminded about the importance of regular brushing, flossing, and rinsing to foster oral health — the dental trinity. However, knowing what's good to do for my teeth and doing them are two separate things, and the distractions of our consumer society don't help any. In 1989, the first commercial teeth-bleaching product was marketed for use at home, sparking the giant $300 million esthetic dentistry industry. Myriad over-the-counter products are available today, promising those with dingy yellows a chance to recover that pearly white sex appeal again. This is an important issue if you smoke, since you're more likely to have stained teeth than your non-smoking friends. As well, current smokers are more likely to report social limitations because of their teeth, including avoiding laughing, smiling, and even conversing because of the condition of their teeth.[14] But as important as bright smiles and personal confidence may be, teeth whitening does nothing to address the critical issue of oral bacteria and inflammation.[15] It may be possible to remove yellow staining with bleaching or to temporarily cover up halitosis with mints, but bacterial mischief carries on unchallenged if this is the only intervention. Bleaching has no effect on reducing gum disease or on the systemic inflammation that follows, just as whitewashing an unstable fence provides no structural improvement. In fact, the structural integrity of the teeth may be compromised by repeated bleaching treatments. Bleaching has been associated with increased tooth sensitivity and irritation of the gums. Depending on the strength of the peroxide solution used and the duration of treatment, repeated whitening treatments can reduce the fracture resistance of dentin and erode our tooth enamel, especially for those people with pre-existing gum damage and receding gums.[16]

Professional plaque removal and regular, close attention to dental hygiene are proven effective interventions that have been shown to both improve smile quality and reduce inflammation on our blood vessels. In addition to biannual dental reviews, dentists recommend a daily, three-step dental hygiene approach to include brushing, flossing, and using an antimicrobial mouth rinse.

"Oh, please don't tell me how to brush my teeth again. I'm a grown adult!" Or so I was thinking when the hygienist demonstrated proper brushing technique on the cutesy stuffed teddy bear with plastic dentures. But as with any technical skill, it can always be improved upon, even when it comes to brushing your teeth. For example, she demonstrated that gum inflammation can be reduced by applying the side of the brush against the gums with a gentle massaging action to stimulate them. I doubt that I'm the only one with things to learn about brushing. Most of us do a fairly slovenly job of dental care. For optimal oral care each tooth surface needs to be scrubbed at least once a day to remove food debris and bacteria. Using a brush with medium to soft bristles minimizes gum trauma, and replacing your toothbrush every three months is recommended. Electric toothbrushes improve thoroughness, and their expense pays dividends at the dentist's office.

A useful exercise to check your brushing technique is to use plaque-disclosing tablets. The school nurse used to hand out the red-dye pills to us elementary school kids during dental week, to illustrate the need for careful brushing. First, we were given an opportunity to brush in our usual manner. Then we were asked to chew on a dye pill and swish the accumulated saliva around in our mouths for about a minute. In addition to turning our tongues bright scarlet, the red chemical attached to areas of dental plaque on our teeth and demonstrated where we needed to give more attention. Even as a child, it was a very humbling experience to smile in front of the mirror after having just brushed madly, and see a mouthful of red-stained teeth.

Using a fluoride toothpaste helps to strengthen tooth enamel and protect it from the damaging effects of bacterial acid. Remineralization of the tooth enamel is a dynamic process, and fluoride from toothpaste is incorporated into the enamel on exposure, making the teeth less vulnerable to bacterial attack. Careful brushing can reduce the number of bacteria to under 100,000 per tooth. Brushing the tongue is also time well spent, since nearly half of our oral flora are lurking amid the 3000 taste receptors in our mouths. Choose a time of the day when you're not too tired or rushed, so that you can methodically do the job that needs doing, following the adage, "don't rush; brush!"

Flossing does two things for me consistently: it cuts the circulation to my fingers and makes my gums bleed. But with proper technique, I'm reassured, it also reduces dental plaque buildup more effectively than brushing alone. Flossing around each tooth mechanically removes the bacterial biofilm collected over the day and helps reduce plaque accumulation and tooth discolouration. With reduced plaque there is less demineralizing acid available to damage the enamel and gums. My teeth are quite crowded, so flossing has always been a bit of a chore. I particularly hate when the floss gets jammed between the teeth and breaks during attempts to free it, leaving bits of frayed floss hanging there like stringy corn. Using coated floss or dental tape gives some slide action and makes the job easier. As well, the more regularly one flosses, the less painful a process it becomes. Now, if I forget to floss, I really notice the difference and miss that just-been-to-the-dentist feeling.

Using mouthwash may seem like good money down the drain,

but my dental colleagues don't agree. They say that the use of an antimicrobial mouth rinse immediately after flossing helps to delay the recolonization of bacteria on the freshly cleaned tooth surfaces and may have some merit in improving oral health.[17] However, prolonged mouthwash exposure can damage the oral mucosa. There's no need to hold the rinse in your mouth for any longer than the few seconds it takes to swish and spit, as daily use of chlorhexidine mouth rinse following mechanical care has been shown to effectively reduce dental staining and plaque formation.[18] As well, rinsing with water after meals and snacks will help dislodge food debris and reduce bacterial numbers.

With Fear and Trembling

I was six years old and felt so small in that stiff, reclined dental chair, staring up at the bright surgical lamp overhead, the white ceiling beyond, and the trays of metal instruments positioned around me. It was a frightening place for a child, made all the worse by the unfortunate visual similarity between my dentist and Dr. Frankenstein's Igor. Old Dr. Dekkar was a stroke survivor. I can still picture him lurching down the hallway with one leg dragging. Worse still, his demeanour fit his appearance. "No cavities, I hope, young man," he would say, as he chose the mirror and pick from his tray of torture tools to tap over my molars. Needless to say, I was a diligent brusher and was thankfully able to survive such episodes unscathed.

Dentistry has come a long way from those dark days. During a recent root canal, I lounged back and watched *The Matrix* with a DVD headset, nearly oblivious to the work being done. The drilling coincided with Neo's escape from the agents, and the procedure was over before the movie was (I had to go home with a rental of the movie to complete the experience). My children also enjoy their dentist visits — of course, the Game Boy in the waiting room helps, as does the sugar-free gum reward that follows their assessments. The future of dentistry holds even more high-tech promises than just entertainment distraction. A space-aged, new drug delivery system is currently under design, using artificial molars to store sustained-release medication. Featuring a sensor, an electrical timing mechanism, and a valve to gradually dissolve two weeks' worth of medication, IntelliDrug fake teeth may some day take the place of pills, syringes, and inhalers.[19]

Regular dental review can help keep gum disease in check. Dental hygienists can best remove stubborn and hard to reach plaque by a process called scaling. This cleaning of tooth surfaces helps to destabilize bacterial footholds. Periodontal therapy has been shown to enhance healthy tooth surfaces and reduce attachment loss. Serial X-rays can assess areas of pain and estimate amount of bone loss between and around the teeth. Dentists also inspect the tongue, cheeks, and throat for early signs of oral cancer — particularly important for those who smoke. It's ideal to attend the same dental clinic, where your dental records and X-rays can be reviewed as needed. Your dentist can develop a staged, interventional plan and assess progress over time. Periodontal therapy can improve your oral health and thereby improve your vascular function.

Eagle Eyes

Another way to mechanically remove bacteria from the mouth is by eating more fibrous foods. When I was in medical school I had to put in late hours poring over my pathology, biochemistry, and anatomy texts. To keep me focused through the boring bits and to calm my nerves before exams, I got into the habit of eating carrots. I would peel five or six large carrots and cut them into sticks, which I would chomp through over the course of an evening's study. I ate so many carrots, in fact, that my palms turned orange. Not the "you're orange, you idiot" that Dr. Gregory House might comment on, but noticeable, nonetheless. Carrots are rich in the pigment beta-carotene, which gets harmlessly deposited in the skin if eaten in large quantities. In the 1970s, beta-carotene was used as a tanning pill, and advertised as "the tan you take." But people preferred the "Blame it on Rio" bronze tan instead of turning sickly orange, so the product didn't fly. Our body uses beta-carotene to make vitamin A, the night-vision vitamin. To capitalize on this phenomenon, British pilots were encouraged to eat carrots to improve their night vision for bombing precision during the Second World War, and supposedly, like mine, their palms turned orange. The Nazis thought they'd do one better. Instead of using beta-carotene to improve night vision, they fed their pilots straight vitamin A tablets instead. This way, they thought, they would bypass the liver conversion step and be that much more efficient. As a result, their palms didn't turn orange. Unfortunately for the Germans, however, vitamin A is toxic to the liver in high doses and can be fatal. The rest is military history.

Mindless snacking can easily be transformed into smart snacking. The ingesting part can remain brainless, but some thoughtful planning beforehand can make all the difference to help reduce dental plaque (and minimize excess calories). For example, I chop up one carrot, one stalk of celery, a four-inch-long portion of English cucumber, and add a small handful of pea pods into a four-cup plastic container before I head out for work every morning. I keep the box in the work fridge and munch on its contents in the afternoon and often in the car on my drive home. It fills my stomach to curb the afternoon munchies and provides an opportunity to mechanically remove plaque from dental surfaces. The fibre and complex carbohydrates aren't usable by oral bacteria to make sticky footholds, so it's a double whammy effect on reducing plaque and bacterial glue all in the same move. My smoking patients tell me that eating crunchy snacks helps them deal with their nicotine cravings, offering a hand-mouth activity without perpetuating their addiction. Who knows, maybe you'll be able to reduce the number of cigarettes you smoke while you reduce your dental plaque!

Sugar is what oral bacteria want, so reducing dietary simple sugars is the key step to reducing oral bacterial numbers and minimizing tooth decay. The problem is that sugar is ubiquitous. As one dieter complained, "if you are what you eat, then I'm cheap, fast, and easy!" Never before have we had such abundance of sugar calories made so affordable. Everywhere you turn there's sugar, added for its flavour, texture, and preserving power. If you read the labels on processed food you will find that they all contain some form of sugar: dextrose, glucose, fructose, maltose, lactose, sorbitol, mannitol, malt, or all of the above if you're in the Twinkie section.

Bacteria metabolize sugar to make energy so they can become self-realized. As a by-product they produce lactic acid, which removes the protective enamel from our teeth, rendering them susceptible to decay. The longer our teeth are in contact with acid the more damage results. Minimizing sticky sweets, such as toffee, gum, and raisins, gives bacteria less opportunity to attach to tooth surfaces and makes the dental cleanup an easier job. Soft drinks represent the number-one source of added sugar in the North American diet, with 50 grams of sugar, or the equivalent to ten spoons per can — that's nearly a 125 ml or a quarter-cup of sugar! One way to offset this oral sugar load is to drink the pop with a meal. At least then, the increased saliva produced for chewing and digesting the meal helps neutralize the bacterial acids and wash the bacteria from our mouths to the hydrochloric acid pit in our stomachs. Even better is to skip the pop altogether and train yourself to drink water with meals and rinse with water between snacks.

As well, rather than going for the glucose rush come snack time, consider a dairy choice instead. Dairy products, like milk and cheese, contain calcium in a very available form, which can counteract the calcium loss occurring with tooth decay. Casein, the major protein in milk, allows replacement of minerals back into the teeth. Studies are currently underway to investigate the role of casein gum in reducing dental cavities in children. Here are some snack-substitution ideas that will help improve oral health rather than accelerate dental decay.

Try This ...	Instead of This ...
carrot sticks	Kit Kat chocolate bar
apple chunks	apple juice
celery and peanut butter	peanut brittle
grapes	raisins

baked potato or salad	french fries
fresh berries	candy
trail mix with nuts	cookies or dougnuts
plain yogurt or cheese	ice cream or sweetened yogurt
pretzels	potato chips
milk	soft drink

Peter's Whitewash

I rarely ever saw Peter's teeth. He always had that Clint Eastwood–pained look on his face, which wrinkled further when he smiled. Like many of my smoking patients, he was self-conscious about his dentition.

"When's the last time you saw your dentist?" I inquired.

"I go if there's a problem, and my teeth haven't bothered me for years. Sure, they're a little dingy, so I was going to get some whitening strips, but that's about all," he said defensively.

"Your teeth need more attention than just whitening," I suggested. "Besides, whitewashing the stucco isn't going to keep the walls from falling down."

"I haven't had any 'walls' fall out yet," Peter argued. "And that's even with rugby, bantam hockey, and growing up with two older brothers," he stated proudly, showing me his yellow, but intact, front teeth.

"Well, if you want to keep your teeth where they belong and help reduce your heart risks, it would be wise to get physical with dental plaque," I said. "Dentists recommend a three-step approach: daily brushing, flossing, and rinsing, as a start."

Peter shrugged. "Sounds like work to me."

"Five minutes is all," I countered. "And if you want to get a jackrabbit start at removing the dental plaque, set up an appointment with your dentist this week. A healthy mouth, a healthy heart."

6

GUT REACTION

"Stressed" Test

Peter was pacing in front of the window when I walked into the exercise lab. His steps were few since he was tethered to the treadmill by a series of electrodes that connected him to our monitor.

"That time of the year so soon?" I asked.

He nodded a "yes" and sat down beside the treadmill so my nurse could record a baseline blood pressure measurement.

Peter had been coming in for annual treadmill testing for the last number of years as part of the motor vehicle requirement for maintenance of his Class 1 driver's licence. He was tapping his foot nervously as he sat waiting for me to get my papers organized and begin the test. I glanced down at his freshly shaved chest and joked, "Not to worry now. It'll grow back long before beach season begins."

"Not too sure how I'm going to do today," Peter said. "I haven't really been doing much lately. And you know, I'm not one for winter sports. It's just *too cold* outside! And I've also been fighting a bit of a cold these past two weeks. I didn't sleep well last night on account of all the sneezing and coughing," he complained, stepping up onto the treadmill platform.

"No excuses now," I answered as I started the belt. "You did nine minutes last year without much difficulty. Six minutes is all the motor vehicle regulation requires. You'll do just fine. It's all under four miles per hour, after all."

"Well, with this belly, that's plenty fast," Peter complained, patting his protuberant abdomen. "I know I've got to work this thing off. Probably this spring," he said as he got into his stride.

"How are you planning to lose the paunch come spring?" I inquired, knowing full well that such vague statements rarely, if ever, come to fruition.

"Not sure … I'll decide … in the spring," he replied in telegraph fashion as the treadmill increased in speed and incline.

"That reminds me of the Mark Twainism: 'why put off to tomorrow what you can put off to the day after tomorrow!'" I mused. "But when it comes to reining in the midriff, I wouldn't procrastinate," I cautioned. "Abdominal fat is bad news. It's a key cause of inflammation in our bodies, and our heart and blood vessels hate it."[1]

Planet Girth

Big bellies have come to town, and it's not just Santa's. Over half of our population is overweight, and nearly a third obese.[2] We are a lipid-laden nation, burning up the world's precious resources to feed our insatiable appetites, and consuming far more food than we are willing to burn in our sedentary lives of comfort. Even school kids are waddling around with muffin tops and butterball bottoms. But the concern here is far from that of cosmetics or body image; this is a critical *health* issue. Obesity kills. Despite the fact that nearly half of the world's population still goes to bed hungry, malnutrition is no longer the top gun in the Grim Reaper's arsenal. Obesity has become the most prevalent nutritional disorder in the world, outstripping undernutrition and infectious diseases as the most significant cause of illness and death on the globe.[3]

From a heart perspective, not all fat collections are of equal concern. Excess padding over the rump, thighs, arms, or neck might reduce one's modelling opportunities, but won't affect the heart nearly as much as adipose over the abdominals. More so than fat anywhere else on the body, abdominal fat stores are associated with increased risk of vascular disease.[4] This realization that excess tummy harms the ticker is fairly new stuff for most of us. Fat cells aren't simply docile energy storage sites, sitting there quietly and minding their own business. Depending on the size of the fat cells and their location within our bodies, they can become quite active metabolically.

If fat cells get large enough, they can be transformed from meek and mild Clark Kent storage cells to Superfat, able to leap tall buildings in a single bound! Well, maybe not. But when fat accumulation crosses a certain threshold, the cells become like glandular tissue and ooze metabolically active hormones into our circulation. If these fat cells happen to be located in the midst of a rich blood supply, as our abdominal stores are, then the secreted proteins readily cross into our blood vessels and get distributed throughout the body. The hormones secreted by transformed fat cells are called adipokines (pronounced "add-dip-po-kines"), derived from adipose, or fat, and kinesis or movement. These messenger proteins allow fat cells to "talk" to other cells. But it's not just idle chitchat about the weather or what to wear to the party tonight. The adipokines secreted from abdominal fat cells activate the white blood cells in circulation and turn on our inflammatory machinery. Like the bacterial toxins from our mouths, these messenger proteins cause vascular damage by creating an inflammatory reaction within the walls of our blood vessels. It is by way of inflammation that abdominal obesity can both initiate and accelerate vascular injury, leading to an increased risk of heart attack and stroke. So if we want to reduce our risk of developing vascular disease, we have to join the battle of the bulge.

The Deadly Quartet

This association between abdominal fat and heart disease isn't a new one. Back in 1947, the French physician Dr. Jean Vague observed that his portly patients were more likely to develop heart attacks than those who retained their svelte figures. But it wasn't until the last twenty years that the details of this relationship have been uncovered. As it turns out, no belly's an island. Abdominal fat doesn't cause vascular inflammation in isolation, but, rather, as part of a larger full-body conspiracy. In the 1980s, investigators noticed that high blood pressure, abnormal cholesterol levels, and elevated blood sugar all seemed to congregate in people with increased abdominal fat. Since it was unknown at the time why these clinical factors occurred together, the grouping was referred to as Syndrome X, to maintain the allure of mystery. Most of us didn't take much notice of the association at the time, but now, with the rising tide of expanding midriffs sweeping the nation, the medical community is paying attention; the audience is listening.

Thanks to the efforts of countless research groups, the interacting mechanisms of these seemingly distinct clinical parameters to produce vascular disease has been worked out. The puzzle pieces have been assembled into a disease entity that we now call the Metabolic Syndrome. Today's medical students are expected to memorize the complex and elegant pathways linking abdominal fat to alterations in sugar metabolism, cholesterol levels, and blood pressure, and to recognize the red flag of heart risk when they occur together. On their own, each of the Metabolic Syndrome factors, such as high blood pressure or abnormal cholesterol levels, increases the risk of heart disease. But in combination, there's serious trouble. Population studies have shown that people with the Metabolic Syndrome have two to three times the risk for developing heart artery disease or stroke, compared to those without the syndrome.[5] In light of the effect of the Metabolic Syndrome on vascular risk, we need to make adjustments to our estimation of 10-year risk scores (see Chapter 1).

If a patient meets the diagnostic criteria for Metabolic Syndrome, we have to take this into account. To arrive at a more accurate 10-year risk estimate of heart attack, we need to double their Framingham risk score. And if you're still smoking, that's double trouble!

Each of the clinical parameters has a well-defined threshold that can easily be measured by your family physician. To be diagnosed as having the Metabolic Syndrome, you need to have at least three of these parameters in the abnormal range.[6] It's estimated that upwards of 25 percent of the North American population makes this cut, and over 40 percent in those over sixty years of age. Since the centrepiece of the Metabolic Syndrome is abdominal fat, the place to start to see if the diagnosis might fit is to measure your waist circumference. So, enough sitting and reading! It's time for action, to get your circulation circulating. Let's measure your waist circumference. Relax, it'll be fun. And besides, no one's around to view your measurements.

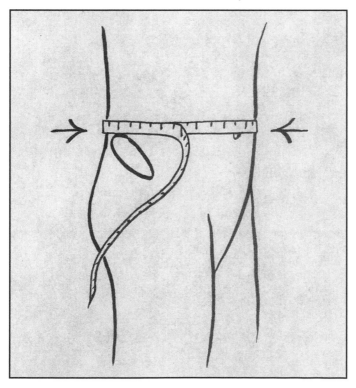

Figure 6.2: Waist circumference measurement.

1. You'll need a cloth tape measure — the paper ones rip too easily, and the metal ones don't bend well and are too cold against the skin.

2. Bare your abdomen so there's no constricting clothing.

3. Loosely wrap the tape measure around your midriff at the level of your belly button. The tape measure shouldn't be pulled so tight that it indents or marks the skin.

4. Breathe easily and take the measurement after you gently breathe out your air. (Sucking in your gut with a big breath is cheating).

5. Record your number. If it's over 102 cm (40 inches) for men or 88 cm (35 inches) for women, you've got some work ahead of you to turn off the fat-induced inflammatory response. If your number is under the threshold, it will be important to keep it there.

Abnormal waist circumference values will vary somewhat depending on gender and ethnic background. But like the measurement of blood pressure, waist circumference is a biological variable. It's not an all-or-none thing. The risk of developing heart disease increases steadily with the increasing degree of girth, and if we're not careful, the Metabolic Syndrome quartet will play our tune. Likewise, keeping abdominal fat to a minimum will help reduce our risk of heart disease and stroke.[7] Having said this, we don't need to hold up the sacred six-pack as our goal. Unlike the chiselled abs so often displayed on magazines at the grocery check-out, heart health is well within reach for most of us.

Metabolic Syndrome's Deadly Quartet

Clinical Parameters	Diagnostic Criteria
Abdominal fat	Increased waist circumference in men > 102 cm (40 inches); in women > 88 cm (35 inches)
Elevated blood pressure (BP)	High BP > 130/85 mmHg
Elevated blood sugar level	High fasting blood sugar level > 6.1 mmol/L
Abnormal blood fat level	High triglyceride > 1.7 mmol/L Low "good" high-density cholesterol (HDL) < 1 men and < 1.3 women

Energy Crisis

"Why is our society suffering from the paunch plague?" you might ask. Why is it that everywhere we look today, belts are buried and six-packs profoundly padded? Energy imbalance has been cited by many as the fundamental problem in this age of excess: too much energy into our bodies in the form of calorie-dense food; and too few calories burned by our bodies, due to inactivity. Few would argue that the overabundance of high-calorie, low-quality food is a central factor that has added considerably to our ever-increasing waistlines. Everywhere you look there's a fast food outlet or some oversized billboard advertising some "full meal deal," where you can "get two combos for just $2 more!" It's an energy crisis, but in reverse. It's not a shortage in fuel availability, as we endured during the 1970s when we were encouraged to car-pool in four-cylinder Japanese compacts. Now the problem is a surplus of energy (of the edible variety), due to a vast and ever-expanding cornucopia of fast-food items begging our attention throughout the day. Never before have so many North Americans eaten out on such a regular basis (and on such base fare) and dined at home so seldom. In time, what is popular becomes the norm, and what is considered normal eventually gets stamped as being good and right. Dietary reform is sorely needed to save us from our excess. Unfortunately, the much-needed return to "slow food" hasn't yet picked up much steam in these parts.

If we were pitching hay bales or laying bricks for a job all day, we might be able to stay ahead of the excess energy we so readily consume. But on average, we Canadians lead sedentary, energy-conserving lives. The computer age has encouraged our desk-bound lifestyles, exercising the mind but leaving the body wanting. Once lean hunters and gatherers on the land, we've been reduced to hunting and pecking on the keyboard. For some of us, the only stretch we get is reaching for the ctrl-alt-delete keys. While typing on a word processor may sometimes seem like tough slogging, in terms of energy output, it's a negligible calorie burner. Automated creature comforts surround us; so much so that one has to make a concerted effort these days to burn any calories above the basal metabolic rate. If I don't plan a walk or exercise session during the day, I can readily settle into a low-output existence myself. Thanks to my garage door opener, automatic transmission, elevator at work, email correspondence, and light clapper, I can easily save all my food energy for frontal fat, if I so choose.

Clandestine Calories

A considerable contribution to our excess energy intake is related to how calories are cleverly hidden. In the 1970s, food manufacturers invented a sweetener called high-fructose corn syrup, which was cheaper and sweeter than plain sugar. Often referred to as modified corn syrup on food labels, this manufactured marvel has found its way into a staggering number of foods, increasing the calorie content of innocent-appearing products such as ketchup, pasta sauce, cookies, cereal, commercial white bread, and soft drinks. As a result, it's easy to consume a sizeable number of calories and not even know you've done it. Most people don't even consider beverages as a source of calories, but they are indeed, and liquid calories are among the worst that exist — empty calories with little or no accompanying nutritional value, just a whole lot of fat-building potential. The average percentage of calories from North American beverage consumption exceeds 25 percent of our daily intake. Sugar-sweetened soft drinks and juices have been implicated as a leading culprit behind the childhood obesity epidemic we're currently facing.

Calorie Content of Selected Beverages

Beverage	"Empty" Calories
Coca-Cola Classic (355 ml can)	155
Glass of wine	170
Apple juice drink (473 ml bottle)	225
Beer (355 ml)	240
Mixed-alcohol drink	300+
Starbucks Frappuccino	470
Super Big Gulp	800

"How is it possible to knock back a 44-ounce Super Big Gulp containing 800 calories and still feel hungry?" I asked my teenage son. He answered with a smile and opened the fridge to look for something to eat. Hollow legs, maybe, but, as it turns out, liquid calories don't play by the same rules as do those from solid food. This is because the mechanisms controlling hunger and thirst are quite different from each other. Our sense of thirst is triggered by water balance. When we take a drink and our body cells have reached a certain water threshold, our thirst is quenched, and we reach for another handful of salted peanuts, setting the whole process in motion once more. By contrast, our sense of hunger relates to the contents of our stomachs and the release of the hunger hormone, ghrelin. When our stomach and intestines get stretched from eating food, ghrelin levels drop, and our hunger pangs diminish. But liquids pass through our gastrointestinal tract quickly and don't do enough stretching to turn off release of the hunger hormone. As a result, our brain doesn't get the message that we've just drunk a meal's worth of calories, even if we have. Since fluid calories don't suppress the hunger response, drinking calorie-dense beverages won't slow us down from eating the same amount of food with our meals. As a result, alcoholic beverages, pop, and fruit juices end up simply adding more calories to our calorie-laden feasts. But there is some good news: since liquid calories don't contribute to feelings of satiety, cutting back on them won't make you feel deprived. Eating calories in the form of solid food and quenching our thirst with water helps our brains keep things straight and balance the energy books better.

Haste Makes Waist

As important as underactivity and overconsumption may be in producing abdominal fat storage, they are not the only culprits causing weight gain. Stressful living makes us prone to storing abdominal fat. Dieters repeatedly complain that "no matter how little I eat and how much I exercise, I keep gaining weight." Of course, there's a grain of salt needed here. The ins and outs of calorie consumption are inherently difficult to estimate. Studies have shown that some people with weight problems suffer from significant caloric misperceptions; underestimating their daily food consumption by over 1,000 calories, while simultaneously overestimating their daily activity by over 250 calories — a miscalculation of over 1,200 calories. Considering that 3,500 calories make a pound, it wouldn't take many mathematical errors of this magnitude to satisfy Shylock's pound of flesh request. But while the complaints of some dieters may be exaggerated, there *is* more to the problem of waist gain than simple energy imbalance.

Stress makes us prone to storing abdominal fat and, since typical North Americans lead fast-paced, time-sensitive, crammed-full lives, we face significant psychological stress throughout the day. From the moment the alarm rings in the morning to the time we crash at night, we're on the run, making haste, and, as it turns out, making waist. Job stress accounts for some of this stress. Work environments, where psychological demands are high and freedom to make decisions low, are associated with an increased risk of heart attacks. As mentioned in Chapter 4, psychological stress can fire up our fight-or-flight response just as readily as any physical danger. When we're under the gun, stress hormones are released into circulation, readying our bodies for action. The stress hormone cortisol is responsible for much of this action, including storing energy in the form of belly fat. So it's not just chowing down on comfort food that pads our pot. When we get frazzled from traffic backups or an interrupted night's sleep, cortisol release intentionally lays down fat in and around our abdominal organs, eventually pressing our belts to a looser notch. Smoking also increases cortisol levels and may explain why some smokers are more prone to getting fat laid down on the midriff than elsewhere on their bodies. This refuelling phenomenon is intended to ensure a ready supply of energy in preparation for future shock. The abdomen is the target locale, since the rich blood supply allows for easy access to mobilize the fat if the need arises. But of course, since the threats we experience are predominately psychological, and not physical in nature, the stored fat sits on our tummies and accumulates, eventually playing havoc with our hearts and our health. The obvious solution is to decrease the release of cortisol by reducing the stress in our lives. You know — slow down and make the morning last, smell the roses, keep the Sabbath, get your eight hours of sleep, stop smoking, and just chill. As the old saying goes, "When in a hole, the first thing to do is to stop digging." Unfortunately, when it comes to stress, most of us are compulsive diggers.

The AB Riot

We are obsessed with the muscular midriff. All eyes are riveted on the likes of Jennifer Lopez and Janet Jackson, sporting coveted sculpted stomachs as a distraction from their distinct lack of singing ability. And what a societal paradox: never before has our fashion culture been so fixated on promoting the well-developed abdomen as the symbol of attractiveness, and never before have we as a nation buried our abdominals so deeply in layers of fat. Body sculpting is a billion-dollar industry, and the well-developed rectus abdominus muscles have become its insignia of physical success. But just because someone may be able to grate cheese on their rippling midsection doesn't guarantee they're healthy. Steroid poppers can achieve the look, but be unable to complete a five-mile fun run to save their lives. A well-developed midriff is not an indicator of aerobic capacity. In fact, the sacred six-pack is probably a better marker of self-idolatry than physical fitness. Like Narcissus, the handsome youth from Greek mythology, who was condemned to fall in love with his own reflection, the ab worshippers are doing as much or more for the mirror industry than for their long-term health.

The good news for us mere mortals is that we don't have to boast a washboard abdominal musculature to be healthy. While chiseled abs might be considered the current badge of health by the marketers of the so-called beauty industry, they are unnecessary to achieve and enjoy heart health. This is important to understand, since many of my patients figure that if they can't achieve Brad Pitt abs, why should they bother with weight control at all? Nothing could be further from the truth. From a cardiovascular vantage point, it's not about superficial appearance; vascular health is worked out on a deeper plane. We need to concern ourselves more with turning off the inflammatory machinery that's injuring our blood vessels. To accomplish this we need to trim down some, yes. But instead of crunching out a thousand sit-ups a day, we can get out from under the grip of Metabolic Syndrome by focusing on modest weight control. Studies indicate that reducing our body weight by as little as 5 percent can pay marked health dividends. It's the relative amount of weight loss that stops the fat-induced inflammatory process. And for more good news: abdominal fat is easier to mobilize and lose than fat located elsewhere on our bodies. The risk of diabetes, high blood pressure, and joint disease all plummet with just a moderate reduction in fat excess, achieved with some attention to our dietary eating pattern and twenty minutes of daily exercise. Looking buff is nice for the beach, but if it's heart health you're after, there's no need to climb that mountain. Slim down the stomach, by all means, but then move past the navel gazing and on to healthier things.

No Quick Fix

We live in the express age of microwave popcorn, TV meals, minute rice, instant breakfasts, instant pudding, insta-banking, instantaneous news coverage, immediate service, high-speed Internet, and high-stakes online gambling. So when it comes to weight control, it's natural that we would want to have it pronto as well. Many feel that they should be able to achieve their ideal body weight cheaply, quickly, and easily, like getting a Big Mac at the drive-thru window. But when it comes to reducing abdominal fat, there is no shortcut. It took years to put on the extra weight, and it will take a gradual process to reverse it as well; a whole new lifestyle needs to be adopted, including an increase in activity level and a reduction in empty calorie consumption. Of course, so-called health marketers disagree, as they try to convince us that *their* diet program or exercise gadget will be the ticket to a beautiful body.

In the realm of diet and weight control, the gap between scientific evidence and popular opinion is a vast chasm.[8] In my clinic, I routinely get peppered with questions on weight loss. Here are some examples.

What about the all tomato diet? I have a friend who lost thirty-six pounds after just six weeks.

Talk to the family of the late Brazilian supermodel Carolina Reston, who died at the heart-breaking age of twenty-one. A victim of the modelling industry's perverse desire for ultrathin, she was a stunning size zero model who suffered from anorexia. According to reports, she stayed clear of most food, except for tomatoes, and died of malnutrition. Extreme dietary restrictions like this are extremely dangerous. Sure, if you cut out one or more food groups you'll lose weight, but it's far from healthy weight loss. Our bodies depend upon a variety of nutrients for optimal function, exemplified by Canada's Food Guide. Fad diets are so named because they show brief, flickering promise and then prove to have no value, or even worse, are shown to be dangerous to health. The golden diet that's going to melt away your excess weight in two weeks is a marketing ploy. It's better to put the magazine back on the shelf and wheel the grocery cart over to the produce section.

Are there pills that can help you lose weight?

Adolf Hitler thought so. Records from the Second World War indicate that he received injections of uppers in the form of amphetamines, with the expressed purpose of helping him stay slim, so he wouldn't take on the Winston Churchill look. In addition to increasing metabolic rate and burning calories, amphetamines are "power drugs" that reduce fatigue, heighten aggression, and diminish human warmth and empathy — not a good choice for a tyrant. Diet pills have had a tough time keeping their place on the pharmacy shelf. Take Fen-phen, for example. This combo drug of fenfluramine and phentermine was an anti-obesity drug that had to be withdrawn from the market after reports surfaced linking the pill to heart-valve disease. With over 50,000 product liability lawsuits filed by alleged victims, totalling over $14 billion, it's going to be some time before this drug sees the light of day again. Of course, this hasn't stopped the pharmaceutical industry from pursuing other medical possibilities. Currently available weight-loss drugs have been shown to assist patients with modest weight loss if taken over several months and up to a year. However, since their long-term safety profile is unclear, they are generally only used for those suffering from life-threatening obesity issues. While numerous other drugs promising magic weight loss are under investigation, the answer for reducing abdominal fat and the resultant heart disease risk won't be found in a pill bottle.

Isn't there some new fat vaccine that can suppress appetite?

This is already old news. The Cystos obesity vaccine was designed to knock out the hunger hormone ghrelin, a small protein that regulates appetite. It was based on the theory that if this appetite gremlin was inhibited, it would make sticking to a diet easier. While a successful vaccine against obesity would be worth billions in our predominately overweight society, this one didn't survive the initial testing, due to disappointing side effects. Now, I'm all for the development of weight-control aids, but such innovations won't remove the need for proven, effective, healthy eating patterns and regular exercise for achieving and maintaining heart health.

I watched a program on TV last night that discussed how surgery is going to cure the obesity epidemic.

Thank you, Oprah. Certainly, surgery does play a role in the management of obese patients: morbidly obese patients, that is, people suffering from the detrimental health effects of their obesity, including heart disease, diabetes, sleep apnea, and orthopaedic issues. There are a number of surgical procedures, termed *bariatric* surgery, that have been developed to aid weight loss for those dying of problems caused by their fat excess. This is not to be confused with cosmetic removal of fat, such as liposuction. Bariatric surgery involves the modification of the gastrointestinal tract to reduce its ability to absorb nutrients. These procedures include reducing the size of the stomach with stapling or banding, removing a portion of the stomach, or bypassing the stomach completely. Studies have shown that significant, life-saving weight loss can be achieved with these approaches. However, there remain some risks and complications with these operations. As well, bariatric surgery doesn't address the lifestyle issues that set the stage for the weight gain in the first place, nor does a surgical approach magically remove the emotional baggage that often accompanies obesity. Nonetheless, bariatric surgery can be lifesaving and offer those debilitated by obesity a jump start on a new and healthier life. But if you want a cure with surgical steel, then get in line. Given the numbers currently waiting for operating time, we'll likely be living in *Star Trek: The Next Generation* before your name comes up for surgery.

Every time I quit smoking I end up gaining weight. Isn't it better to smoke and stay thin than stop and gain all that weight?

Although nicotine can increase our metabolic rate and burn about 10 calories per cigarette, smoking is an inefficient, expensive, and unhealthy weight-control method. Terminal cancer is a far more effective weight-loss remedy, but no health solution, either. Excess fat on the abdomen can be harmful on the heart and blood vessels, but it's small potatoes next to cigarette smoking. Weight loss in and of itself cannot be our only goal, and you don't need to be thin to win the heart health game. To help counter weight gain during smoking cessation, it's doubly important for the reformed smoker to have well-established, healthy eating patterns and to make healthy food choices. This is because cigarette craving and hunger for food can invoke similar sensations, rendering the newly reformed smoker continuously hungry and liable to eat food to quench the nicotine cravings.

Spinning Wheels

"How shall I spend my summer vacation? Hmm. Let me count the ways." I had several options to choose from. I was asked to speak at a week-long conference in Whistler (nice place, but rich food and golf aren't my preferred mix). There was the old boys backcountry hiking expedition in Kananaskis country (beautiful scenery, but I'm set against the idea of being served up at a bear banquet). We had a gift certificate for tennis lessons at our community recreation centre (reasonable exercise, but chasing balls gone wild can be humiliating). Last, there was the prospect of heading to a bed and breakfast for some rest and relaxation. This option attracted me the most, but my brother arrived on the scene with something else in mind. He was turning the fragile fifty and wanted to mark his big day in a memorable way.

"How about we bike the Icefield Parkway in July?" he asked. "Come on, it'll be really neat!" (Did I mention he was turning fifty?)

I know the Parkway well. It's probably the most beautiful stretch of highway on the planet, joining Lake Louise to Jasper National Park in the pristine Rockies.

"It sounds nice. You got access to a couple of motorbikes we can use?" I asked, imagining myself straddling a hog and cruising down the carefree highway, *Easy Rider* style.

"Not motorbike, just plain bike, as in bicycle. You know, using leg power, your own steam!" he corrected me, with endearing impatience.

"No thanks," sprung immediately to mind, but he was insistent, and so my vacation choice was made.

There are generally three types of cyclists seen on the Icefield Parkway. The first is the back-to-nature group. They're the ones with the matching tie-dyed tops and bottoms, slogging along slowly with fully loaded ten-speeds. Under the weight of their sleeping bags, tent, cooler, cook stove, granola, and clothing for all seasons, they look like the Beverly Hillbillies. But because they're completely self-sufficient and camp en route, they earn the moniker "rough-and-tough bikers."

The second type includes the impediment-free, high-tech racers. These neoprene-suited hardbodies, with matching helmets, are sleek and streamlined, speeding past like some alien invasion. Using ultralight racing bikes, complete with aero bars and camelbacks, they ride the entire 240 kilometres in a single day. Of course, they're not self-sufficient, as is the rough-and-tough cyclist type. One can see their entourage; an entire motorcade support team in convoy style, complete with on-site personal trainers, a gourmet chef, and a masseuse to see to their every whim and fancy. But they look good and are thus referred to as the "buff bikers."

Now, being neither rough-and-tough nor particularly buff, my brother and I joined the ranks of the third type of cyclists — the mature and sophisticated "past-the-primers" (did I mention that he was turning fifty?). This meant that we had nothing to prove to anyone. Since neither speed nor self-sufficiency was expected, we could just relax and take in the scenery, and call a taxi if trouble arose. So we spread the trip out over five days and stayed at hotels along the route. This way, our panniers were lightly packed with just a sweater and rain shell, as well as some assorted instant energy gels and water. Ours was the most civilized approach to biking, unless, of course, you have a motorcycle.

Not wanting to get weighed down with heavy foodstuffs, we decided to limit ourselves to two meals per day: breakfast before embarking from the hotel in the morning, and dinner after arriving at the next hotel in the evening. Who needs a bulky lunch or a heavy snack pack when you've got mountains to climb? Perhaps the trip would get me in shape. I figured that with the restricted calorie consumption and six plus hours of solid biking per day, I'd resemble some kind of Greek god by week's end. Needless to say, I was surprised to feel my bike shorts fitting *more* snugly as the trip progressed. But I wasn't just imagining the increase in ab padding. When I stood on the scale after our trip was completed, my weight had actually gone up! "Huh?" I said, as intelligently as I could. How is it that my weight increased, with only two meals a day and with thousands of calories burned along the roadside (especially on the steep, hilly bits)? Why, after such a physical expedition, did I look less like Hercules and more like Buddha?

"Elementary, My Dear Watson"

I sheepishly explained the situation to one of my dietician colleagues, over a small salad and glass of water. She reminded me of two weight-loss myths that were likely at play on my bike tour, and that steer countless dieters down the wrong path. The first myth she debunked was the need for calorie *restriction* to enjoy weight control. "Doesn't diet mean calorie restriction?" I asked innocently. Not so, I learned. A better definition is "eating with intention." So many diets are based on limiting the number of calories, since starvation is considered an absolute requirement for many who embark on a weight-loss regimen. Weight Watchers' programs, for example, revolve around calorie counting, reducing the attributes of food to merely its energy value. Every meal and snack is broken down into the number of calories it contains, and dieters are encouraged to record every food item on elaborate charts, from the bowl of muesli in the morning to the Melba toast at dinner. But accounting for every calorie with endless reams of math has to be dizzying. You can't blame subscribers of calorie-restricted diets for eventually getting frustrated, ditching their program, flashing on Dr. Phil, and having a bag of Lays with a full-calorie Pepsi.

Spreading out our calorie consumption over the course of the day is more likely to meet our physiological needs and less likely to result in midriff storage than going hungry all day and then piling it on at dinner. Of course, there is some merit to knowing something about calorie content, particularly if you're considering ordering a St. Louis Hardee's Megaburger, which boasts two one-third-pound slabs of Angus beef, four strips of bacon, three slices of cheese, slathered in mayonnaise on a buttered bun, and all told containing some 1,420 calories (nearly a full day's caloric needs). And, yes, portion control is important. When it comes to weight control, those who eat seconds are often the first losers. But there's got to be more to life than trying to meticulously balance the body's energy equation. Rather than fixating on this tedious numbers game to restrict calories consumed, we need to pay some attention to when we eat. Our eating patterns and, in particular, the timing of our calorie consumption play an important role in weight control. As it turns out, it's not just playing jazz that depends on timing. If we can eat quality foods spaced throughout the day, we'll go a long way towards reducing weight concerns.

Despite what some diet evangelists might preach, calories aren't the incarnation of evil. The Metabolic Syndrome isn't caused by consuming timely calories, but by over-consuming unnecessary calories. Our bodies need energy in the form of calories to perform life-sustaining activities. Even when we're just sitting quietly reading *Heidi*, we still need energy for lung respiration, heart contraction, and liver and kidney activities. This basal metabolic rate can require between 1,000 and 2,000 calories per day, depending on body size and composition. Our brains, for example, need a continual supply of energy, day and night. Being the control centre of the body, the noodle gets what it wants; even if it means that other parts of the body go without. So when my brother and I were starving ourselves each afternoon on our bike trip, slogging past the Athabasca Glacier, our brains didn't suffer for lack of energy (not that they were being overly taxed in any way). Where did the calories come from if we weren't eating until dinnertime, 60 kilometres of pedalling away? Not to worry, our bodies will find calories for maintaining vital function. But you're not going to like how the body acquires the energy. "If there's a will there's a way," is fine, but doesn't mean the way will foster health.

Calorie restriction is stressful on our bodies, and when the body is under stress, the stress hormone, cortisol, gets liberally secreted. One of the many functions of this stress hormone is energy mobilization. If no food energy is available, cortisol digs deep and finds the needed calories for brain and vital organ functioning by breaking down less vital tissues in your body. Calorie restriction is a prime example of taking from Peter to pay Paul. This dismantling process is called catabolism (pronounced "ka-*tab*-o-lism"). Some may tell you to not let your worries eat you up, and they're right. Catabolism is a bit like self-cannibalism. Stress does eat us up, quite literally. And the hard news is that the location where cortisol does its deconstruction business isn't the fat stores that we'd love to see eaten away. The flesh that gets hit the hardest by cortisol catabolism is our muscles. This is because muscle is high maintenance, luxury tissue, always wanting more calories, more exercise, more stretching, more massage, and more trips to Europe. Fat tissue, by contrast, avoids cortisol's consuming fire, since it requires little energy to be maintained and is content to just sit there and be fat. So, given the chance, the stress hormone devours our muscle tissue to liberate the needed energy that our brains and vital organs demand. Not surprisingly, bodybuilders avoid calorie restriction like the plague.

The additional problem with calorie restriction is what follows when you cave in to your hunger pangs. After my brother and I reached our day's destination, we made a beeline to the hotel restaurant and ate our way through the evening. We had worked hard, after all, and felt that we deserved our just desserts. But the problem with binge eating (even after a lengthy workout) is that too many calories are made available over a short period of time. The body responds with the evolutionary survival mechanism of storing it away in preparation for the next famine. So, although we burned lots of calories biking around mountain passes, we overshot our energy needs when we rested. The cortisol that was breaking down our muscle tissue for needed energy by day, was now storing up the excess food calories as abdominal fat by night. It was a double whammy for weight gain.

The old adage "to lengthen thy life, lessen thy meals" needs some qualification. Lessen the *amount* of a meal, sure, but don't lessen the *number* of meals. Contrary to diet dogma, if you want to reduce abdominal fat (and we do), it pays to eat more frequently. If we scrimp on calories during the day, our bodies are forced to break down muscle, and if we binge eat at night, our bodies are forced to store the excess as more fat. So, rather than skipping meals or binge eating (as we did on our bike trip), it's important to spread out the calories over the course of the day. Ideally, we should eat every two to three hours. That means, for an average waking day we need six to eight meals — small meals. Or we should keep with the three squares and add in three to five snacks, interspersed between them. If we follow this eating pattern, we won't be limiting our body's access to needed fuel nor will we overload the system with a motherlode of calories that it doesn't need, both of which can foster weight gain.

Mom said, "Eat breakfast, because it's the most important meal of the day." Well, for all her nagging, she was right on this point. Studies have confirmed that those who don't eat breakfast are more likely to suffer from weight excess. Eating breakfast is the key weight-control strategy to increase metabolism and is central to most successful weight-control programs. If we don't *break* the *fast* then the body automatically switches into survival mode: breaking down precious, fat-burning muscle for needed calories and slowing metabolism to conserve energy. Starting off the day with breakfast on board tells our body, "Relax, will you? There's no sign of any famine on the horizon, and here are some calories to prove it, so just leave my puny muscles alone!" Front-loading the day's calories gives the body a chance to burn them as it carries out our whims and wishes. If we keep in mind the wise words of Adele Davis, "eat breakfast like a king, lunch like a prince, and dinner like a pauper," we'll more likely be able to rein in our abs.

Too Much of a Good Thing

Extreme sports have never been so popular. It seems that every weekend Edmonton is host to some endurance event or another. It's a triathlon, biathlon, marathon, or ultra-marathon that's blocking traffic. Never before has this planet seen so many endurance competitors. Over 90,000 runners apply annually to take part in the New York City Marathon. In contrast to the original 127 participants in 1970, when it began, over 30,000 athletes now cross the finish line at this world's largest marathon. Even the Grande Cache Death Race, with its gruelling 125-kilometre course, spanning three mountain summits, continues to attract over 1,000 wannabe superheroes every year. And while the health benefits of exercise are well-documented and substantial, they begin to wane with such extreme feats of exertion. But, that being said, most endurance athletes compete first and foremost for the love of their sport. I didn't run the Boston Marathon because I thought it was the best thing for my heart. For me, it was a mountain I needed to climb, as I was recovering from my stroke. The world's oldest and most prestigious marathon race was my rehabilitation ticket. I needed to prove to myself that I could do it: I ran because I could run, not because I needed to for health's sake. Recovering from a heart attack or stroke does not by any stretch of the imagination require such gruelling physical feats.

Not to say that our summer bike trip through the mountains was as extreme as running a marathon or completing a triathlon, but for us it was extreme enough. Spending six to eight hours biking up and down mountain terrain is stressful for the body and amounts to over-exercise. This type of physical stress also liberates cortisol, which may provide further explanation as to why I gained girth on my epic excursion. I had stress-hormone release for two reasons: lack of lunch and ponderous pedalling. As for weight control that week, it was a cortisol double jeopardy.

In the realm of weight control, the mistake many people make is to overdo it on the cardio machines. They have images of sleek Kenyan marathoners and figure long-distance exercise is the only way to get in shape. But hours of low-intensity stair-climbing or plodding along on the treadmill is inefficient fat-burning exercise. Part of the problem with prolonged heavy exertion is the stress response, with release of cortisol. After about a golden hour of exercise, the naturally present anabolic hormones, like testosterone, which assist in the building up of muscle tissue, get overrun by rising stress-hormone levels. Once cortisol levels take over, you can say goodbye to further muscle building. That's why most bodybuilders are careful to limit their workout time to reduce cortisol release. Some also use anabolic steroids, the polar opposite of cortisol, to help them get ripped.

"Well, why is muscle so important? I don't want to look like Arnold Schwarzenegger. I just want to get in shape!"

If getting in shape means getting rid of unwanted fat around the midriff, then it's time to get to know your muscles. Despite what the flashy magazines displayed at the grocery check-out might say, fat doesn't just melt away. Fat needs to be metabolized and broken down into usable work energy, and it's within muscle cells, with their countless, energy-consuming, contractile proteins, where fat gets burned. Those who have less muscle, have less opportunity get rid of fat. As well, your metabolic rate is directly dependent on the amount of lean tissue on your frame, and specifically, the amount of muscle you have. The more muscle you have, the higher your metabolic rate. That means that the exercised hardbody burns more calories during the after-dinner card game than the sedentary softy. As we age, we begin to lose muscle. It's estimated that every decade beyond age thirty, we lose about 10 percent of our muscle mass. This muscle loss means that we arrive at a lower metabolic rate. Unless we maintain our muscle mass, it becomes harder for our aging bodies to burn calories and more difficult to lose weight.

Putting Legs on Weight Management

The value of weightlifting for weight control was made apparent to me last winter when I broke my collarbone skiing. It's curious how a tiny bone, the size of your dinner fork, can so quickly become the centre of the universe. You wouldn't know how important the collarbone is in supporting so many movements and tasks until you've broken it. With only one arm, everything became a chore, especially since it was my dominant right arm. Dressing, driving, brushing my teeth, and even typing were physical feats, accomplished only with care and cursing. Needless to say, my exercise routine needed modification. Jogging was out; the bouncing up and down was too painful. I tried aqua-jogging, but nearly drowned (there's a good reason you don't see many one-armed swimmers). I needed an exercise routine that I could do without using my upper body; one that would help me stay in shape while I waited for my collarbone to heal.

So I took up with the universal machine at my gym, focusing on leg exercises. I felt kind of silly going there with my arm in a sling, but since most flock to the treadmill and elliptical machines, the weight machines were usually free for me to quietly experiment with. I worked out a schedule of leg exercises, comprising leg press, extensions, calf curls, squats, and lunges. I chose three or four exercises for a given workout, which I stuck to three or four times a week. I did ten repetitions of each exercise to make a set, and three sets in a given workout. I was done in less than half an hour, leaving extra time for the hot shower (my favourite part of exercising). After six months of this routine — leg weights three times a week, in addition to my daily walking with our dog — my collar bone was less painful and I was able to re-introduce some upper body exercises. During the recovery time, I did lose some arm and chest muscle (although no one seemed to notice, since there wasn't much there in the first place). But I maintained my leg musculature and, most importantly, I didn't gain an ounce of fat on my abdomen.

Resistance exercise in the form of weightlifting is considered by many exercise experts to be the most efficient means of burning calories. The calorie consumption is thought to occur:

- during the exercise itself, especially if large muscle groups (like those in the legs) are exercised;
- during the twenty-four hours that follow, as your body recovers from the workout and repairs the micro-damage incurred; and
- by adding to the amount of lean body tissue on your body and increasing your resting metabolic rate, the energy burn keeps going, even while you sleep.

Beyond weight control, maintaining our muscle mass is an important determinant in maintaining our functional independence as we age. The weak and infirm are destined to spend their golden years in a nursing home.

The lessons that I learned from my ski injury were the following:

- Lifting weights loses weight. Resistance exercise is effective for weight management.
- Leg muscles are big. Exercising larger muscle groups is more efficient than pumping up the puny ones. Large muscles, like those in the legs, consume more fat in less time.
- Skiing a black diamond run as your last run of the day is folly.

Next Summer Vacation

I would make a few changes if I were to plan a long-distance biking trip through the Rockies again, particularly if abdominal fat was a concern. First, I would pack lots of food to comfortably meet my daily energy needs, spacing meals and snacks every two to three hours (heavy on the fresh fruit and veggies, and with a complete embargo on sickly sweet gels!). Second, I would get my daily exercise by taking an hour-long alpine hike, both before checking out of the morning hotel and again after arriving at the evening destination. That way I would maximize the fresh air exposure and keep my metabolism humming. And third, I'd ditch my touring bicycle and borrow a Honda Goldwing 750 in order to bike in style.

7

CORE CURRICULUM

In Technology We Trust

"Congratulations, you made it!" I announced, reducing the treadmill speed to give Peter a chance to cool down. His daughter looked almost as relieved as Peter when he finished the stress test, intact.

"How was it?" Peter gasped. "Do you see any problems?" he panted.

"Not to worry," I tried to reassure him. "The test looks fine. There's no indirect evidence of any blood flow problem to the heart. And since you did nine minutes instead of the mandatory six, the Motor Vehicles Branch will be more than happy to continue your Class 1 driver's licence," I declared with a thumbs-up sign.

"Do you think I need an angiogram, Doc?" Peter asked as he sat down to rest, not registering any sign of reassurance from my positive pronouncements.

"No," I answered calmly. "We don't do angiograms without just cause. Based on your test today, I don't see any reason to put you through the potential dangers of invasive testing," I further tried to reassure him, as the nurse brought him a glass of water and a towel.

"But can we really trust the treadmill results?" he asked as he downed the water and motioned for a second. "My brother had a stress test, too, and it didn't stop him from dying of a heart attack." He spoke with a bitter tone and a worried look.

"Yes, you're right," I agreed. "This test isn't a guarantee that heart trouble won't come knocking. But neither is undergoing an angiogram, or getting a CT or MRI image taken of your heart. Midas Muffler might give out guarantees, but when it comes to the heart, there are no warranty papers. Medical tests are useful in that they can give us a snapshot of your heart's status, but they don't give us infallible predictions about health and disease, and they do nothing to slow down the disease process."

"So we do nothing?" he asked with a look of frustration.

"If only I were a surgeon, then I could *do* things and get some respect around here," I joked. "Keeping your blood pressure under control, your weight in check, and getting you clear of the nicotine curse are hardly 'doing nothing.' Addressing these things will go a long way in reducing your risks for heart disease and stroke. Putting you through a bunch of unnecessary high-tech tests is like rearranging the deck chairs on the *Titanic*."

"So you think I'm going down with my ship?" Peter asked, dejected.

"Not yet, but you are in dangerous waters," I cautioned. "Let me suggest how you might navigate to safety." I pulled out my PLAC diagram yet again. "The angiogram can tell us how narrowed the heart arteries have become, but it doesn't give us a complete picture of the problem going on inside the blood vessels." I pointed to number (4) Cholesterol Core on the diagram below (see figure 7.1), and said, "Heart attacks occur when this core area of cholesterol breaks open, which can happen even before there's much noticeable narrowing seen on the angiogram. More tests aren't going to tell us anything we don't already know. It's clear from your Framingham Risk Score that you're still at high risk for vascular disease. To help reduce this risk, we need to address this cholesterol core while there's still the opportunity."

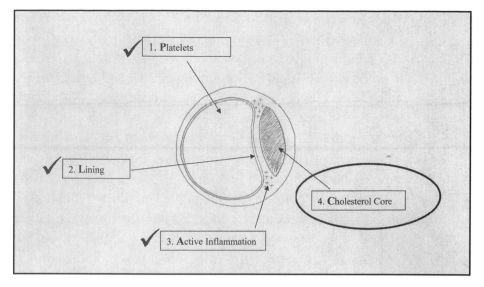

Figure 7.1: Cholesterol core.

The Gruelling Disease

Despite the mammoth advances in medicine over the past few decades, atherosclerosis still accounts for more deaths in North America than any other disease. So, instead of just praying to the god of modern medicine for a magical cure, it may be worthwhile taking some steps of our own to address the serious problem of vascular disease. The term *atherosclerosis* comes from two Greek words that we medics attached together to help us sound intelligent. The first is *athera*, which means "gruel" or "porridge" and provides the visual for what cholesterol deposits look like within the walls of our blood vessels. The second Greek word is *sclerosis*, which means "hardened"; this is what a diseased blood vessel specimen feels like in the pathology lab. Taken together, they mean "hard porridge" — something like when you arrive home after work to find the breakfast dishes piled up by the sink, still unwashed by your teenage son who promised to clean them, and now the porridge is stuck on the cereal bowls like cement. If your heart arteries look like your porridge bowl, then come on down, you've got atherosclerosis and can take your chances playing *The Price Is Right*: behind door number one is heart disease; door number two, stroke; and number three, dead on arrival — good luck!

"Why the food descriptors?" some might wonder. Well, pathologists are the ones largely responsible for the naming of diseases. They don't get out much and need some creative outlet, so they use nomenclature as a sort of morbid game. One of their favourite pastimes is choosing food names to describe their specimens, such as bread-and-butter pericarditis, honeycomb lung, and nutmeg liver (not particularly appetizing, especially if you've seen the pickled specimens). But disease isn't pretty, and atherosclerosis is one hard porridge that even Oliver Twist would think twice about before asking for "more please, sir."

The first time I came face to face with this vascular gruel was during my training as a surgical assistant. An elderly patient had come into the emergency department complaining of severe pain in the lower abdomen and back regions. He was ashen grey when I saw him and was found to have a life-threatening tear in his aorta, the largest blood vessel in the body. (Where's the little dike boy when you need him?) He went straight to the operating room for emergency surgery.

"What causes the tear in the first place?" I asked, with puppy dog eagerness, as the surgeon prepared to make his incision. "Pay attention and you'll have a chance to see firsthand," he growled, giving me two large metal retractors to hold back the abdominal contents.

As I did my best to hold the retractors in place and keep the aorta in view, the surgeon found the tear. He then placed two metal clamps across the damaged vessel, one above and one below the tear, so he could replace it with a tube graft. When the clamps were snapped in place, pinching off the aorta, they made an audible crunching noise, like broken glass underfoot.

"It sounds more like bone than a blood vessel," I remarked, as I accidently let go of one of the retractors. Not amused, he repositioned the tool and showed me the torn portion of the vessel. It was covered in white calcium deposits and pockmarked with ulcerated sores, like a severe case of teenage acne (not wanting to mix metaphors, I kept this observation to myself).

"There's your answer," he said. "This is why the aorta tore." He pointed to the raised grey and yellow bumps spotting the surface of the diseased vessel and added dryly, "Hardened porridge."

Pipeline to the Heart

Thanks to angiography, we don't have to rely on the direct inspection of blood vessels to make the diagnosis of atherosclerosis. Developed decades ago, angiography is an invasive procedure that has allowed doctors to view the size and contour of blood vessels, located pretty much any place in the body, without surgical exploration. Angiography is another example of two Greek words pasted together: *angio* refers to "blood vessel" (pronounced "Angie," as in Mick Jagger's tune, and "Oh," as in "Oh, get on with it already!"), and *graphy*, "let's take a look see." Sometimes the procedure is called catheterization, which simply means "inserting a tube." If the tube in question is a bladder catheter, for draining urine, it can be done simply enough (assuming a cooperative and continent subject), but when it comes to vascular catheterization, it takes highly specialized equipment and a skilled team to perform it safely with reliable results.

Vascular catheterization (angiography) involves placement of a catheter or small plastic hollow tube into a blood vessel, which can then be threaded under X-ray guidance to any vascular location under scrutiny. When opaque dye is injected into these carefully placed tubes, the arteries are visible by X-ray imaging and resemble the branches of a tree, with a larger trunk dividing into smaller side branches and eventually twigs. When the tubes are filled with the dye, images of the arteries are captured so we can closely analyze the arteries for the presence of atherosclerotic narrowings. If meals are rich and exercise plans are exorcised, cholesterol deposits can grow into the blood vessel centre and deform the regular, round shape that we see during angiography. The more narrowed a blood vessel is, the more likely it will cause symptoms. An hourglass indentation of the vessel's inner diameter, or lumen, typically signifies the presence of a large coronary plaque. In angiospeak, a significant narrowing of a coronary artery is defined as a plaque occupying 70 percent or more of the vessel diameter. Coronary narrowings of this degree can limit the flow of blood downstream and can very often produce chest pain (angina) or shortness of breath. Although there's currently some competition from the non-invasive imaging technologies like CT scanning, angiography remains the gold standard for determining the presence and severity of atherosclerotic heart disease.

The application of angiography for heart investigation is credited to a twenty-five-year-old surgical trainee from Germany, by the name of Werner Forssman. It was 1929 when this wannabe cardiologist thought he'd apply what he'd learned in the animal physiology laboratory to human investigations. He made the bold assertion that it would be possible to get access into the beating human heart by using a hollow tube inserted into an arm vein. "Sticking a tube into a living human heart?" his supervisor asked incredulously. "With what, a garden hose?" The trainee answered by holding up a ureteral catheter — a long hollow and flexible tube used to help kidneys drain past obstructing stones. With such a visual retort, his supervisor likely blanched, slammed his fist onto the table, and spit out something along the lines of "@#*# *Dummkopf!! Das ist ein verrucktes idioten Idee!*" (Translated: "Well, my word, that's unconventional.") At that time, of course, the medical community had no experience with ticker tinkering. It was widely agreed that the heart was forbidden territory — a surgical no man's land. Part of the concern was that insertion of a tube into the heart might set off a lethal heart rhythm disturbance (which is certainly a risk of the procedure). The other concerning part was what to do if, indeed, that happened.

His chief said, "heads vill rrrrroll" when young Werner persisted with applying his theory. But Dr. Forssman not only ignored the stern warning of his department chief, he also supposedly tied his nursing assistant to an operating table to prevent her interference with his landmark experiment — on himself. He made an incision into one of his arm veins and inserted the tip of the urinary catheter. To help him guide the tube towards his heart, he used a fluoroscope X-ray camera and rigged up a mirror so he could view the screen. Standing under the fluoroscope camera and peering into the mirror, he threaded the tube up his arm vein, watching the X-ray image as the tip of the tube moved past his shoulder, under his neck, and down into the right side of his heart. Recognizing that this was truly a Kodak moment, he walked upstairs with the catheter tip in his heart, went into the radiology department, and took the confirmatory X-ray picture. He was probably on cloud nine with excitement, because he then eagerly went back to his boss to show him the proof — that it was not only possible to place a catheter in the human heart, but it was also possible to tell the tale. Being true to his word (and a bit of a stick-in-the-mud), his chief fired him on the spot. Nevertheless, in 1956, Dr. Forssman was formally recognized for his contribution to medicine and was awarded the Nobel Prize for his vision and bravado.

Although angiography remains an important investigative tool in medicine, its application today has progressed well beyond mere diagnostics and into the realm of therapeutics. If we see a tight heart artery, plugged with cholesterol plaque, we don't just make note of it, pat the patient's hand, and say "there, there," sympathetically. By no means! Today, we can routinely dilate severely narrowed heart arteries using miniature balloons inserted through the centre of the angiocatheter. The procedure is referred to as angioplasty or blood vessel fix. Where we once relied on bypass surgery, angioplasty now allows us to mechanically improve blood flow to the heart's magnificent muscle, without having to crack the chest, stop the heart, and do all that cutting and pasting that only surgeons love. Some might even say that cardiologists have taken angioplasty too far, overdoing the balloon dilation shtick. And the critics have a point, since, as Mark Twain observed, "to a man with a hammer, everything looks like a nail." But there's more. By way of the same tiny needle poke in the arm that Werner Forssman demonstrated for us in the 1920s, it's not only possible to image the heart arteries or dilate their narrowings, but to deliver medicines into the heart, prop open diseased vessels with metal scaffolding (stents), close unwanted holes within the heart, using umbrella-like devices, and even fix malfunctioning heart valves. It's a staggering array of technological advances, all using angiography as a foundation, and it's growing by the minute.

"How on earth can they do all that?" one might ask. Well, I doubt you picked this book off the shelf to answer that question. But since the topic has been raised, I'll give it a few sentences and begin by having you briefly consider the boat in the bottle phenomenon. That miniature ship won't sail through the bottle neck unscathed, not even with Vaseline smeared on the mast. No, despite what Captain Highliner may have said while in his cups, the miniature ship is inserted through the neck of the bottle in collapsed form. Once it's nicely in place, a string is pulled, the mast and sails unfold, and voila, we have a Cutty Sark preserved in glass. There may be some variations on the theme, but the catheter-based technologies, like angioplasty and stenting, make use of this sort of design. Using cleverly crafted devices that collapse down to nothing, it's possible to insert them into the angiocatheter lumen and thread them to where they're needed, using X-ray guidance. Once in position, the specialist can release them into the blood vessel in expanded form to accomplish their purpose.

I underwent angiography, myself, not long ago. But it wasn't in the do-it-yourself style of Dr. Forssman. "Physician, heal thyself" hadn't crossed my confused mind that day. In fact, I was in no shape to even tell one end of a catheter from another, let alone thread one into my own heart. I still remember looking up at the neurologist's face as he described the problem and the need for an emergency angiogram. "You've got a lot of nose hairs," I considered saying, since my sudden predicament hardly seemed real, and blithe comments seem welcome in dreamland. I had been whisked to the University Hospital by ambulance because I had collapsed face down in the sand and was unable to move my left side. Within brief minutes of arrival, I received the diagnosis of massive stroke.

"Your carotid artery has dissected [torn asunder]," he told me. "The thrombolytic [clot-buster medicine] hasn't worked, so we need to try to open up the vessel with angioplasty." His eyes looked worried and his voice cracked, giving me the unsettling impression that this wasn't going to be routine.

"Yes, of course," I answered. "Do what you can. I'll be right here if you need me or have any questions."

Aside from the brief sting of local anaesthetic used to freeze the skin where the catheter gets inserted, the procedure was painless. Since there are no nerves on the inside of our blood vessels, you don't feel the threading of the catheter, which, in my case, went from the insertion site at my groin, up the inside of my aorta, along my neck artery and into the smaller vascular branches that keep the bats from my belfry. Injection of dye allowed the physicians to locate the carotid artery tear and position two metal stents to tack down the torn blood vessel segment, repairing the artery from the inside. After the procedure, I was taken up to the neurological intensive care unit to recover from the day's excitement. The nurse there asked me some routine questions to check my level of consciousness: "What's your name? Where are you? What day is it?" No problem there; I scored three for three. And then came the real test: the neurologist asked me to squeeze his fingers with both of my hands.

"Hey!" I said. "Will you look at that! Return of the prodigal limb. I can move my paralyzed arm and make a fist!"

The angioplasty procedure successfully opened my blocked blood vessel and allowed me to enjoy a remarkable recovery. I walked out of the hospital three days later.

Thanks to the ingenuity of medical pioneers like Dr. Forssman and the many skilled physicians who perform such invasive procedures, patients like me can safely undergo lifesaving interventions and return to their lives intact. Being able to walk out of the hospital without the need of a walker or cane, embrace each of my boys using both of my arms, and tell them how I love them so in ungarbled words was a gift of immeasurable magnitude, for which I will be ever grateful.

Vascular Icebergs

People often joke that they can "feel the ol' arteries a pluggin' up" when they're eating a high-fat meal. It's become a bit of a morbid compliment to the cook these days; "great dinner Auntie Jean, I'll check in for my quadruple bypass after dessert!" And while it's true that fat and cholesterol absorbed from a meal can impair the normal functioning of our blood vessels within hours of ingestion, the plugging part isn't caused by cholesterol circulating in our bloodstream; that trouble originates deep within the walls of our blood vessels. If you liken the vascular wall to that of your house, cholesterol deposits aren't located on the beige-painted inside surfaces or fresco wallpaper; they lie underneath the dry wall and behind the pink insulation.

Cholesterol gets into our vascular walls by first circulating around the body, packaged in protein carriers called lipoproteins. The most notorious example is the low-density lipoprotein, or LDL cholesterol particle. These fatty monsters have been identified as the ringleaders in cardiovascular crimes, and for good reason; LDL cholesterol not only injures the lining of our blood vessels, but it cuts to the core. LDL cholesterol undergoes a biochemical reaction called oxidation.[1] It's similar to what's happening right now on the rocker panels of your unwashed Camry, thanks to the salt trucks. Oxidized metal is rust. When LDL cholesterol gets oxidized it becomes like the Tasmanian devil and sets off an inflammatory reaction under the vascular surface. Smoking cigarettes accelerates this LDL cholesterol oxidation, illustrating one of the many ways in which nicotine addiction is harmful.

Our trusty white cells are called into action and attempt to calm the cholesterol chaos by the only means they know — eating (sound familiar?). The problem with this approach is that white cells can't dismantle the cholesterol they've eaten. We can make it in our livers, convert it to different hormones, if need be, and even excrete it with our bile, but our bodies have no way of breaking down cholesterol.

Over time, the white cells get transformed into what we call foam cells. These porky, fat-filled cholesterol containers are good for nothing and end up accumulating within the walls of our arteries. That's why it's so important to limit dietary intake of cholesterol; once it's on board, it's staying on board and going down with the ship.[2] As it turns out, our well-intended white cells are unknowingly on a suicide mission. They stuff themselves with cholesterol until it kills them — similar to what you might see at an all-you-can-eat buffet. In time, these dead foam cells coalesce into an ever-growing, cholesterol plaque that litters the long and winding road of our blood vessels. From this hiding place, cholesterol collections bide their time for a break-and-enter opportunity, typically waiting for the most inopportune time to spew their contents into circulation and cause a heart attack or stroke.

"Why not dilate all the coronary plaques, even if they aren't causing symptoms?" worried people ask me, wishing to avert such an event.

"If it ain't broke, don't fix it" satisfies some, but for the keeners who want to know the real deal, I break down and tell them the truth. Balloon angioplasty is wonderful for dealing with symptomatic coronary artery disease, but indiscriminate use of angioplasty balloon dilation does nothing to reduce the risk of future heart attacks.[3] We can make the "after" angiogram pictures look pretty and line our wallets aplenty, but if our aim is to somehow reduce this burgeoning burden of vascular disease that has us swamped and sinking, we've done very little. The studies are in: preventative angioplasties haven't made the least dent on heart attack rates. We need to somehow get to the core of the problem and not just monkey with the vascular complexion.

Using miniature ultrasound cameras inserted inside a catheter and threaded into the heart arteries, we can see these cholesterol collections before they cause their mischief. Because ultrasound penetrates tissue planes it allows us to look below the blood vessel surface. So, unlike angiography, ultrasound gives us a glimpse of the various layers of the vessel wall, like looking at a sedimentary rock stratum. And what we've learned is that cholesterol plaques don't just grow inwards, making the blood vessel hole opening narrowed; vascular plaques also grow outward, expanding the size of the blood vessel.[4] In fact, they preferentially grow outward, sometimes with very little effect on the shape of the blood vessel hole or lumen. It's not until the plaque accumulates within the blood vessel wall that the lumen begins to shrink and the blood flow gets reduced. If you think of a blood vessel like an old-fashioned doughnut, angiography just shows us the middle — the Timbit part. So, if the plaque is deep in the cake of the doughnut and growing outward like some kind of cruller, it will be missed by angiography. Like an iceberg that sits three quarters below the ocean's surface, the cholesterol core of an atherosclerotic plaque lies largely under the inner surface of our blood vessels. And like an iceberg, just because you can't see the hidden portion, doesn't mean it's not dangerous. In fact, the vascular plaques that cause the so-called mild indentations we see during angiography are the ones most likely to cause heart attacks. Unless cholesterol levels are reined in, these 20 to 30 percent narrowings can be quite unstable and prone to rupture, and squishing a stent over them does nothing to stop the problem — believe me, it's been tried.[5]

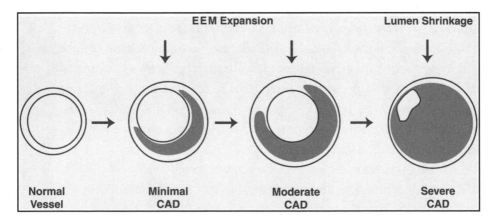

Figure 7.2: Glagov diagram showing the progression of plaque accumulation in the coronary artery wall with initial expansion of the external elastic membrane (EEM) and later the shrinkage of the blood vessel lumen. Courtesy of S. Glagov, E. Weisenberg, and C.K. Zarins, "Coronary Artery Plaque Progression." *New England Journal of Medicine* 316 (1987): 1371.

If we're doing angiography under the illusion of preventing disease, we're deluding ourselves; we don't see the full plaque burden and we're likely going to gloss over the site of the future heart attack. So, as important as revascularization procedures are in reducing symptoms, it's only the severe and symptomatic coronary plaques that require mechanical dilation. Flattening cholesterol plaques against the blood vessel wall does nothing to slow the disease process itself; atherosclerosis unrelentlessly marches on, placing an ever-tightening stranglehold on our hearts. Like time and tides, cholesterol deposits wait for no one. We need to stabilize the cholesterol core before it breaks open and cuts off critical blood flow to our hearts and heads. To do this most effectively, we need to reduce the amount of cholesterol in the plaque from the inside out.

An Inside Job

Fortunately, such a remedy is at hand. No, it's not giving up eating (although that's a thought). And no, it's not another pharmaceutical creation, or something you buy in boxes or bags with ribbons and tags. No, the most efficient means of removing dangerous cholesterol build-up from our arteries is already in our possession. It's a cholesterol-lowering remedy that was built in when we were knit together. Why, thank you, Mother Nature! The remedy is called the reverse transport mechanism for cholesterol. It works by backpedalling the flow of cholesterol away from our blood vessels. The wee vehicle that makes this transportation possible is called HDL, which stands for high density lipoprotein. Affectionately referred to as the *good* cholesterol protein, HDL binds onto the cholesterol it finds messing with our blood vessels and shuttles it back to our livers. From there, the heart-attack-inducing stuff gets processed into something more useful for our body, like growth hormone for muscle building, or it gets excreted altogether. HDL steadily grows in size as it makes this pilgrimage from peripheral tissue to liver, grabbing onto more cholesterol as it goes. But like our car's transmission that has many forward gears and only one reverse, the HDL transport system gets quickly overwhelmed by the lipid-laden lives we lead, where cholesterol is continually pushed forward from our plates and into our blood vessels.

As in most things, from firing neurons to material wealth, the distribution of HDL is not equal among humankind. Men tend to have lower levels of HDL, as do those who sit around a lot, eat Oreos, or smoke (another way nicotine's doing you wrong). And when it comes to predicting heart attack risk, HDL is like a crystal ball. The Framingham study showed that for a given level of LDL, or bad, cholesterol in the body, the risk of developing heart disease varied wildly, depending on the HDL level.[6] Those who had the lowest levels had ten times the risk of dying of a heart attack, as compared with those who had the highest HDL levels.[7] But fortunately for us HDL-underachievers, our good cholesterol levels aren't carved in stone. With some intentional steps, it's possible to bolster our HDL levels, no matter where they may currently sit, and stabilize our cholesterol plaques, no matter where they're currently sitting.

Raise a Little HDL

Once upon a time, in a land far, far away, there lived a healthy, happy people, who were free of all vascular ailments because they had discovered the elixir of life: an easy-to-swallow, sugar-coated, inexpensive pill that raised their HDL levels beautifully, and without any undesirable side effects. Unfortunately, this isn't our story. We live in the throes of vascular calamity, and although we've recognized HDL as an important player in improving health, we have no simple way of optimizing HDL levels. So, take a deep breath in, let it out slowly, and allow me tell you about the real-life challenges of getting it up (HDL, that is).

To date, there is only one medication that's been shown to be reliable, effective, and safe in doing the job. Some swear by it; others swear if it's mentioned. It's a B vitamin called niacin, and here's the scoop. The year was 1914, and the place was the Rankin penal colony in South Carolina. "I have an announcement!" bellowed the guard, as the inmates put down their work. "There's a doctor here from the government." The prisoners peered over each others shoulders to get a view of their visitor. "He's looking for volunteers to take part in a human experiment," the guard barked, and the convicts' curiosity was replaced by concern. "And all of you are going to sign up. Now back to work!" he yelled, as the pained prisoners shuffled back to their menial tasks.

Dr. Joseph Goldberger was the U.S. Surgeon General at the time and had already climbed the career ladder successfully, but wanted to clinch his prominence for posterity's sake (in medical circles that usually means making the centerfold in some prestigious medical journal). He saw the opportunity with a disease called pellagra — a horrible ailment that begins with a nasty skin condition, involving the sun-exposed areas, and progresses to diarrhea, dementia, and eventually death (usually in that order). No one knew what caused it at the time, but since it looked at bit like leprosy and most commonly affected corn consumers, most assumed it was an infectious disease. But Dr. Goldberger had a different theory. He was an epidemiologist, which means that he went to school for a really, really long time, studying disease patterns in populations, so he had plenty of time to ponder things such as the cause of pellagra. He reckoned that since this skin affliction hit mainly the impoverished, malnutrition was a likely culprit. To prove it, he needed some "volunteers." A penal colony was a good place to look, since it's easier to control the dietary intake of inmates, and also because they're just so darn eager to oblige. To prove if imbalanced nutrition caused pellagra, he put them on an all-corn diet. His menu may have included such things as corn chips, with cream of corn for dipping; corn chowder, with all-you-can eat corn biscuits; a side of corn-on-the-cob smothered in corn syrup; and popcorn for dessert (not bad, if you don't mind the corn). And he was right. His careful study clearly documented the relationship between the corn-restricted diet and the development of pellagra, which he was able to successfully reverse afterwards by providing his incarcerated guinea pigs a more balanced diet.

In 1937, it was discovered that the missing ingredient for the pellagra prisoners was vitamin B_3, naturally found in a variety of plant (green vegetables, tomatoes, beans) and animal sources (meat and fish). So it was called the pellagra-preventing factor. Today, we call it niacin, which not only prevents pellagra, but increases the good HDL cholesterol levels by a whopping 10 to 30 percent. The kicker is that many cannot tolerate the side effects of niacin supplementation. Niacin causes release of prostaglandins, setting off an unpleasant, itchy, prickly, flushing sensation, which most people find quite disagreeable. My menopausal patients even claim that their time-of-life symptoms pale by comparison to the flushing of niacin. There is a slow-release formulation of niacin, called Niaspan that may reduce the flushing side effect to some degree.

A few highly motivated individuals don't seem to be too bothered by niacin's flush, but their motivation isn't so much heart health as a fear of the law. They erroneously believe that niacin can flush traces of street drugs, like marijuana, out of their system so they can evade detection. It doesn't work, of course; niacin flushes the skin royally, but does nothing to flush drug levels. Besides, when it comes to marijuana, it's better to listen to the sage advice of our infamous Olympian snowboarder, Ross Rebagliati — if you're going for gold, don't inhale. So, despite the fact that the flushing side effects can be limited by taking Aspirin beforehand, or by eating food concurrently, most of my patients stay clear of niacin.

"Is that the only medicine you've got? Isn't there some other pill I can take to raise my HDL levels?" ask the drug obsessed. Other than niacin, drug therapy has been very disappointing on this front. There have been some valiant attempts though. Torcetrapib was the promised wonder drug; the Neo of the cholesterol Matrix, that was to raise good cholesterol levels to record heights. But it turned out to be as much of a failure as its unpronounceable name, and was ditched because of unanticipated liver toxicity.[8] Drugs from the fibrate and statin classes have been touted to raise HDL, but their contributions for this purpose have been meagre, at best. But even though the pharmacy may be of limited utility in raising HDL levels, it's still possible to get it up there. In fact, there are a variety of other ways that can be very effective, indeed, including dietary adjustments, limited alcohol consumption, and exercise, or even better, a combination of them all. Some might argue that so-called lifestyle approaches are too hard-won for their minimal HDL-raising effect, but it's important to bear in mind that even small changes in HDL levels can have dramatic benefits for the heart. For every 1 percent rise in HDL cholesterol, the risk of getting a heart attack drops by 1 percent.[9] In addition to cholesterol control, lifestyle manoeuvres, such as physical activity, quitting smoking, and reducing excess fat, are all associated with improved health in general, and heart health in particular. If we want to reduce the risk of heart attack and stroke, it's critical to reverse the flow of cholesterol away from our blood vessels. Even baby steps, in the right direction, will take us a long way along the road to health.

Raising HDL Levels

- moderate aerobic exercise
- mild alcohol consumption
- weight loss
- soluble fibre in the diet
- monounsaturated and polyunsaturated fat in diet instead of trans fatty acids or saturated fat
- omega-3 supplement
- niacin supplement

The French Connection

The French seem to have a good thing going. Using the North American diet as a benchmark, numerous studies have shown that despite their increased intake of fatty foods and wine, the French have a lower incidence of heart disease than us model citizens. According to the statisticians, the French eat an average of 108 grams of saturated fat per day, in contrast to our North American consumption of only 72 grams per day; they eat 60 percent more cheese than we do (it may even be higher than this, since that orange gooey substance we call Cheez Whiz can hardly be compared to any of the 365 French varieties of *real* cheese); the French eat three times the amount of pork we do and four times the amount of butter! And after all that sinning, only 83 citizens per 100,000 succumb to heart attacks annually, while we North Americans suffer over 230 annual deaths per 100,000 from our fat-fearing mopey crew. The injustice is enough to make anyone west of the English Channel feel like *Les Miserables*![10]

Chief Inspector Clouseau lays out the evidence on his bureau, poring over it with his magnifying glass. "Neuw let me see here, what could explain this most fascinating phenomenon of French food supremacy: the antioxidants? Could it be the higher HDL levels? Perhaps the phenolics in the wine? Hmm … they are all under suspicion. I just don't kneauw." But before epiphany can strike, Cato, his trusty sidekick, jumps him from the ceiling fan. "Not neuw Cato, yeu fewl! This iz your employer speaking … I am calling off the attack!"

There are numerous theories that attempt to explain this French Paradox. The diet-conscious figure it's the natural fats used in French cooking, rather than the heavy reliance on trans fatty acids, as in our North American diet. Another viewpoint is that the French have fewer heart attacks because they eat more slowly and masticate their food properly, chewing each mouthful twenty-five times, rather than wolfing down their dinner before pulling out from the Wendy's window. The psychological perspective considers the suggestion that the French don't view their food as the enemy, but delight in the presentation and mouth-watering aroma of their meals, and savour each morsel. Those in the fit and firm group remind us that Europeans in general, and perhaps the French in particular, walk and bike everywhere, from the Louvre to the Eiffel tower, and that their cardioprotection is due to their improved fitness levels. One unusual assertion is that the French are protected from heart disease because they don't shave their armpits, and accrue less blood loss. But when the French are asked why their hearts fare better, they shake their heads and say, "*Mais non, monsieur*, it is, how you say in English … the *joie de vivre!*"

While many of the above theories may have some merit in giving reason for the French connection to heart health (except perhaps the argument about the hairy armpits), the prevailing wisdom figures it's the alcohol consumption.[11] Supposedly, the French drink over 50 percent more alcohol than North Americans. But the benefits aren't felt to be restricted to French Bordeaux or other red wine selections. Sure, red wine has bioflavinoids and antioxidants that protect the heart, but so does unfermented grape juice and raisins. Despite the desires of the wine industry to place health food labels on their bottles of *vin rouge*, it appears that the most important ingredient in red wine for heart protection is the ethanol. So regardless of the form — from *Marilyn Merlot* to *this Bud's for you* — it seems it's the alcohol, not the alcoholic beverage, that provides the cardiovascular benefits. The mechanism is complex and involves alcohol's positive influence on a variety of heart-health parameters, inflammatory markers, blood-clotting proteins, nitric oxide levels, blood-sugar control, and, of course, raising HDL levels.

"Rock on, dude! Like that's just totally awesome news, Doc. Like you're the best. Score me another Silver Bullet! Here's to my HDL, yeah, right on!"

Not so fast. While it's true that population studies have shown a relationship between alcohol consumption and cardiovascular protection, this is no carte blanche for taking another bottle of beer off the wall. The benefits of drinking alcohol occur only at the low end of the consumption scale: somewhere between 7 to 14 grams of alcohol per day, which works out to about one drink for ladies and one to two for the gents.[12] As well, the benefits are relatively transient, lasting for twelve to twenty-four hours. It's the small, regular exposure that's the health ticket, like having a glass of wine with the family meal. Drinking more than this amount quickly negates any benefit, and binge drinking ushers in risk aplenty, including heart rhythm disorders, heart failure, high blood pressure, elevated heart attack risk, stroke, sudden death, cirrhosis of the liver, gastritis, pancreatitis, addiction, depression, increased risk of marital discord, domestic violence, motor-vehicle-accident risk, driving impairment charges, jail time … you see the concern.[13] Take a look at the figure on the next page, showing total mortality plotted against alcohol consumption. It's a J-shaped curve, resembling the Nike swoosh symbol. Using the abstainers as the reference baseline, it shows a lower risk for those who drink one to two drinks per day, but then a marked and brisk increase in risk of death for those who imbibe increasing amounts of alcohol.

The health limits on alcohol aren't anything new. Aristotle said, "one glass for health, two for gaity, three for bitterness, and four for intemperance," which George Carlin updated with the adage, "one tequila, two tequila, three tequila, floor." And then there's Dorothy Parker, with her self-effacing realization: "I like to have a martini / Two at the very most. / After three I'm under the table, / after four I'm under my host."

In light of the suggested benefits, should doctors be advocating alcohol consumption? I think not. I work at an inner city hospital, inundated with patients suffering from alcohol abuse. For a physician, the pressing issue is identifying the problem drinkers and mobilizing resources in the community to help them with their dependency. The vast and serious problems surrounding alcohol consumption in our society need no encouragement. The wine industry would have us believe that abstinence from alcohol is a risk factor for cardiovascular disease, but the current evidence doesn't support this ploy for sales. Some would suggest that if we want to lower our risk of vascular

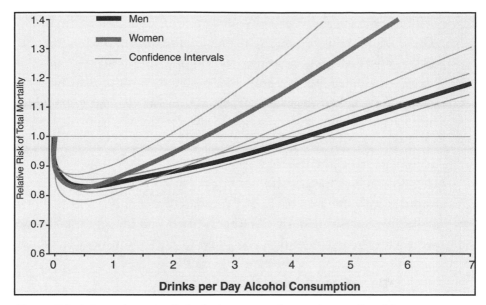

Figure 7.3: J-shaped curve of alcohol consumption and mortality risk. Courtesy of A. Di Castelnuovo, et al., "Alcohol Dosing and Total Mortality in Men and Women: An Updated Meta-Analysis of 34 Prospective Studies." *Archives of Internal Medicine* 166(22) (2006): 2437–45.

disease, we should emulate our European friends and go out and buy a bottle of Beaujolais, a couple of baguettes, a black beret, and sign up for Berlitz lessons. But I hardly think this is necessary. If you do drink alcohol, a one-to-two-per-day exposure should be the limit. Anything more is risky and quickly becomes both unhealthy and dangerous, not to mention fattening (don't forget the calorie content of booze). If you don't drink alcohol currently, you don't have to stock up at Liquor Depot. Teetotalling has its merits — especially if it's green tea with all those antioxidants. And besides, there are plenty of other ways to reduce your risk of vascular disease while you quit smoking.

Survival of the Fittest

Regular exercise raises the good HDL cholesterol level, but it doesn't stop there. The benefits of exercise on the cardiovascular

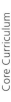

system are many and varied, accounting for the survival of the fittest. Those who live longest on this planet are the ones in the best aerobic shape. Hans Meyer is acclaimed as the first European to climb the snows of Kilimanjiro in 1889. But much more impressive was his guide, Yohana Lauwo, who not only successfully led the great white hunters to the highest point in Africa, but repeated the climb hundreds of times over the next seventy years, living to the honourable age of 125 years. And then there's John Kelly, the many-time winner of the Boston marathon, who continued to run the prestigious race annually into his eighties (I bet I could've beaten his last time, but I pulled my hamstring muscle before the race, and I wasn't used to the weather, or road conditions, and I had forgotten my lucky laces ...).

Benefits of Exercise

- increased longevity
- increased HDL
- lowered atherogenic LDL
- blood pressure control
- blood sugar control
- improved insulin sensitivity
- reduced inflammation
- improved weight control
- improved vascular function

When I crossed the finish line at the Boston Marathon in 2005, I was *really finished* — physically, emotionally, psychosocially, and aromatically. With bleeding toes and salt-caked skin, I staggered over to the food tent for some refreshments, where, to my astonishment, I saw about a dozen finishers (all who had beat my time) sharing their race stories over a cigarette! Smokers ran the marathon? Now, there's a paradox! But it's been clearly demonstrated that physical fitness is an independent predictor of heart health — even independent of smoking.[14] Likewise, sedentary living is an independent predictor of heart attack risk.[15] This is particularly concerning, since if the thought of exercise comes to mind, over 60 percent of Canadians lie down until the feeling goes away. When researchers compared smokers with non-smokers, they found that the "fit" smokers lived longer than the sedentary non-smokers (I don't like to share this bit of info with all my smoking patients because they often take it the wrong way).[16] "This isn't to say that you should keep smoking," I try to sternly emphasize to my patients, with ample hand-waving. Rather, taking part in regular exercise is an excellent way to reduce cardiovascular risks while you quit.

We define cardio-respiratory fitness in terms of how efficiently our bodies use oxygen.[16] The more oxygen our exercising muscles can grab, the more fit we are. The parameter we measure is called VO_2max. Not to be confused with Alberto's VO5 Maxi Hairspray, the physiological parameter, VO_2max, is the gold standard for defining cardio-respiratory fitness. My level was measured when I was trying to improve my personal-best running time. I was not only hooked up to electrodes to monitor my heart rate and rhythm, but I also had to wear a Darth Vader–like breathing contraption that measured how much oxygen I was breathing in, and how much carbon dioxide I was breathing out. Given a taste of my own medicine, I then had to run on a treadmill full tilt, as a couple of exercise technicians in their early twenties egged me on to exhaustion. "Pretty good for an old guy," one muttered as I turned purple and waved them to stop. Although VO_2max is dependent on body size, gender, age, and genetics, it can be improved by exercise. Any improvement is well worth while, since VO_2max levels closely correlate with overall survival.[18]

Directly measuring VO_2max is too cumbersome for day-to-day clinical medicine. I supervise treadmill tests, like the one Peter had that provide an estimate of fitness — close enough for practical purposes. There are even simpler tests that also predict fitness levels with reasonable accuracy that include the six-minute walk test[19] and the Long Corridor Walk Distance (400 metres).[20] Tall, lean, young men do the best, because they can take longer strides and leave less sweat on the track. But all of us should be able to make it around a

Core Curriculum

400-metre track in under six minutes, since risk of death increases if your six-minute walk test distance is under 350 metres.

If exercise is the best medicine (or perhaps a close second behind laughter), how much should we take and how often? The exact dose–response curve for exercise hasn't been as precisely defined as medication doses, but studies suggest that the health benefits resemble a curve, as in the figure on the next page.[21] By plotting health benefits on the vertical axis against energy expenditure on the horizontal axis, you find a direct and positive relationship between energy output and health. As you can see, the steepest portion of the curve is between 800 and 1,400 calories of energy burned per week (or, more precisely, kcal, which stands for kilocalories). This would be comparable to walking between twenty to sixty minutes a day. Although the benefits of regular exercise keep pouring in at higher energy expenditures, the people who get the biggest bang for their butt are the sedentary, who decide to exercise their New Year's resolution and get off the couch. Expending as little as 800 calories per week pays remarkable dividends on your health investment, and the activity doesn't have to be performed all at one time in the day. Similar benefits accrue if walking, for example, is divided into short intervals and accumulated piecemeal through the day. But since the benefits of exercise can't be stored up for a rainy day, it's necessary to take part in physical activity on a daily basis. Being on the high school football team may be a nice memory, but when it comes to your present fitness level, it's forgotten. Exercise, like alcohol consumption, is most protective of your heart when done daily and in moderation. But, unlike alcohol, the sky's the limit; there's no ceiling to the benefits of exercise. So, *just do it*.

When outlining an exercise prescription for patients, I use the FITT acronym for structure: **F**requency, **I**ntensity, **T**ime or duration, and **T**ype of exercise. The ideal frequency of exercise is between three and six times per week (even the physical body needs a break). The safest intensity level to stimulate fitness improvement is in the moderate zone. The recommended time or duration of an exercise session is between twenty and sixty minutes. The type of exercise best suited for health maintenance makes repetitive use of large

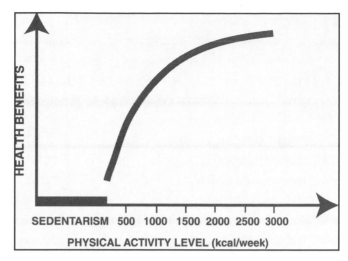

Figure 7.4: Dose response curve for exercise. Courtesy of C. Bouchard, "Physical Inactivity." *Canadian Journal of Cardiology* 15 (Supplement G) (1999): 89G–92G.

HEALTH BENEFITS

SEDENTARISM 500 1000 1500 2000 2500 3000

PHYSICAL ACTIVITY LEVEL (kcal/week)

muscle groups, like walking (my favourite), jogging, swimming, biking, rowing, Thai boxing, and step class. Each exercise session has a certain format for best results: warm-up, main exercise, cool-down, and stretch. The warm-up is to protect your muscles from injury. Those who save time and skip the warm-up often pay big-time with soft-tissue injuries (did I mention that I tore my hamstring muscle?). The cool-down is a mirror image of the warm-up, but this time it's not so much to protect muscles from injury, as to allow your heart an opportunity to slow down gently, and helps protect against heart-rhythm disturbances or rapid drops in blood pressure, both of which can occur if exercise is abruptly stopped.

FITT Parameters	Recommendations
Frequency	3–6 times per week
Intensity	Moderate talk test
Time	20–60 minutes per session
Type	Large muscle use, e.g., walking

Although an exercise prescription is fairly self-explanatory, personal trainers are well worth their wage to help provide instruction on exercise form, so you can get the most benefit out of the activity

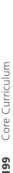

with the least risk of injury. In addition, the only FITT parameter that needs some careful attention is defining exercise intensity. The ancient motto of moderation is a good starting place, and the reasons are twofold.[23] First, it's safer to exercise in the moderate zone, rather than risking an injury. If we think back to the glory days when we were the star 100-metre sprint champion in junior high and try to relive that again without proper training, we're in for trouble — most likely a pulled hamstring muscle (mine still hurts just sitting here). Second, the moderate exercise intensity zone is where we begin to improve our VO$_2$max level. If we're only exercising at a low-intensity, perspiration-free dawdle, we aren't going to give our bodies much of an incentive to improve the oxygen utilization machinery, and it will result in minimal, if any, improvement in our fitness level. One of the uses of stress testing is to help patients with heart disease, define where this moderate intensity level lies for them.[19] Using the maximal heart rate achieved on the treadmill as the basis, we calculate moderate intensity as between 70 and 85 percent of this maximal heart rate. Patients can then exercise into this moderate heart rate zone using a heart-rate monitor, and anticipate the benefits of exercise, without the risks. Another approach to define exercise intensity is to use the so-called talk test, which works like this: low-intensity exercise doesn't affect your ability to gab in the least; moderate-intensity exercise makes it more difficult to talk in long sentences (like reciting Lincoln's Gettysburg Address or Hamlet's "to be or not to be" soliloquy), but you can still talk; and high-intensity exercise reduces any attempt at speech to a telegraph report. So talk it up as you hit the pavement or trails.

Mission Impossible?

"**Good afternoon, Mr. Phelps.** Your mission, Jim, should you decide to accept it, is to disarm a ticking time bomb. It's located in your heart arteries and it's disguised as a cholesterol-filled plaque buried deep within the blood vessel wall. Urgent attention is needed to stabilize the plaque core and prevent mortal ruin. Stabilization can be achieved only by increasing the HDL cholesterol level and reducing the LDL cholesterol level. You will be provided the latest dietary and medicinal suggestions to accomplish this task, but your time will be limited. This message will self-destruct in five seconds."

Here's a dietary must that needs to be clearly understood: *trans fatty acids must be completely eliminated from our diets.* There is no middle ground on this matter. Trans fat (or hydrogenated fat) is a substance that doesn't exist in nature. It's vegetable oil infused with hydrogen under high temperatures. It was designed as the answer to the food manufacturers' wish for a clean-burning, deep-frying oil that's inexpensive, avoids use of the black-listed saturated fats, has an increased shelf life, and expands the taste opportunities for the bored palates of North Americans, like Oreo cookies and Reeses Peanut Butter Cups. Trans fat has found its way into a vast number of convenient processed foodstuffs, including cookies, biscuits, chips, nachos, pies, waffles, breads, fried items (french fries), and movie theatre popcorn. But they're not worth the convenience. Trans fat destabilizes our vascular plaques by increasing the bad LDL cholesterol level and reducing the good HDL level, the polar opposite of what we are trying to achieve. Because trans fatty acids have been identified as accomplices in causing cardiovascular disease, the United States Food and Drug Administration finally required in 2003 that food companies list trans fats on their nutritional labels.[23] Canada followed suit in December 2005. Make a point of looking at these labels some time. Find out which products contain trans fatty acids, and avoid them in the future. Just say "no" and put them back on the grocery shelf or extricate them from your pantry and throw them out — better underfed than dead.[24]

Must number two: identify the enemy. *LDL cholesterol is lethal.* The scientific data to support this assertion is staggering. So, don't undo all your good HDL-raising work, like jogging on the treadmill, by overwhelming the reverse transport system with a package of Twinkies. We need to keep the intake of cholesterol to an absolute minimum, and at the same time choose foods that reduce its absorption.[25]

Raising HDL Through What You Eat

Dietary Intervention	Mechanism	Examples
Fibre (2–10g fibre/day needed to affect cholesterol levels)	Prevents cholesterol absorption in the gastrointestinal tract	Psyllium, oat bran, barley, legumes
Plant stanols/ sterols	Reduces animal cholesterol absorption by competition	Fruits and vegetables; nuts and seeds; soybean oil
Soy protein	Increases LDL cholesterol receptors, removing cholesterol from circulation and from our system	Smoothies with frozen fruit and tofu are an excellent snack option. Avoid dessert tofu because it has added sugar
Poly-unsaturated fat	Increases HDL and reduces LDL (the opposite of trans-fatty acids)	Fish oil, canola oil, olive oil
Mono-unsaturated fat	Increases HDL and reduces LDL (the opposite of trans-fatty acids)	Almonds, walnuts, pecans

You don't have to be a Trappist monk sworn to dietary simplicity to achieve higher HDL and lower LDL levels (although, this isn't a bad idea). The Lyon Heart Study showed that North Americans could dramatically reduce their heart attack risk by adopting a Mediterranean-style cuisine.[26] By using canola oil margarine and olive oil as their main fat source, choosing fresh fish over processed and red meats, including abundant amounts of fruits and vegetables in their meals, and consuming moderate amounts of dairy foods and wine, they reduced their risk of heart attack by an impressive 70 percent. And that's no hardship; I love Grub Med!

Depending on your risk for developing vascular disease, your doctor may recommend a blood test to measure your cholesterol level, and if warranted, medication to help lower the LDL cholesterol level.[27] Today, we have powerful and well-tolerated medicines called statins (e.g., Simvastatin or Zocor) that can help turn off the production of excess cholesterol in the liver and dramatically reduce levels of this vascular monster. Current statin doses reliably reduce LDL cholesterol levels by between 20 and 60 percent, where, with every doubling of the dose, an additional 6 percent reduction is possible.

When Is Fasting Lipid Profile Screening Recommended?

- all men > 40 years and women > 50 years or postmenopausal
- those with diabetes
- current smokers or those who have recently quit (within one year)
- those with high blood pressure
- those with a family history of premature coronary artery disease (first degree male relative < 55 years; female < 65 years)
- those with abdominal obesity (men with waist circumference > 102 cm (40"); women >88 cm (35")

No drug is free of potential side effects. This is true for the statin class of medicines also. Common side effects include muscle cramps, sleep disturbance, nausea, diarrhea, and an elevated liver enzyme blood test (1.5 to 2 times the upper limits of normal). Serious side effects are thankfully rare, but still need to be looked for using a twice-yearly blood test. The serious side effects include hepatitis (liver inflammation), myositis (muscle inflammation), rhabdomyolysis (very rare catastrophic muscle breakdown), and peripheral neuropathy (nerve damage). To help prevent side effects, we tend to choose the lowest effective dosage. If goal LDL levels can't be reached with the statin medicines, or if side effects occur, an additional medicine called Ezetrol can be of use, either alone or in addition to the statin. Ezetrol reduces cholesterol absorption from the intestine and can multiply the benefits when added to a statin. Since it's possible to overwhelm the effect of these medicines by eating high-cholesterol foods, you still need to watch what you eat. Besides, the benefits of nutrition extend beyond cholesterol lowering and include important things like improved plaque stabilization and reduced blood clotting and inflammation.

The two most important parameters from the fasting cholesterol blood test include the ratio (total cholesterol level divided by the HDL cholesterol level) and the LDL cholesterol level. The treatment goals for these parameters are risk dependent. For patients who are at high risk for developing vascular disease (like Peter, for example), aggressive reduction in LDL cholesterol is needed; for patients at a lesser risk, lesser reduction is acceptable. Here are the target cholesterol levels.[28]

Cholesterol Parameter	Low-Risk Patients	Intermediate-Risk Patients	High-Risk Patients
Ratio: Total Cholesterol / HDL Level	< 6.0	< 5.0	< 4.0
LDL Cholesterol (mmol/L)	< 5.0	< 3.5	< 2.0

Peter's Prescriptions

I pulled up Peter's lab results as he was collecting his coat and gym bag. "Your LDL cholesterol is on the high side," I said. "According to last week's fasting blood sample, it measured 4.2 mmol/L. Since you're in the high-risk zone for heart trouble, we need to target a level below 2.0."

Peter shrugged. "Sounds optimistic to me. I'd have to eat like Bugs Bunny to achieve that goal."

"A vegetarian cuisine wouldn't hurt," I agreed. "I'll give you a prescription for a cholesterol-lowering medicine that will get us towards the target. And since the statins work best when we follow a diet low in cholesterol, I'll arrange a consultation with one of our dieticians, as well. She'll steer you down the right grocery aisles."

"How was his good cholesterol, the HDL level?" his daughter inquired.

"Lower than I'd like," I replied. "The HDL level was 0.72, giving us a total cholesterol to HDL Ratio of over five. So, in addition to lowering the LDL cholesterol, I've got a second prescription for you to give the good stuff a boost."

"Not another drug!" Peter complained with an agonized look.

"Better than a drug," I reassured him. "I'll give you an exercise prescription, based on today's treadmill results."

"How safe is it for Dad to exercise?" Peter's daughter asked. "You hear about people keeling over when they're working out — even athletes."

"There is a small risk of heart attack during exercise for everyone," I agreed. "But the risk is highest for those with established heart disease and those who don't exercise regularly. It's the sudden bursts of activity that get people into trouble, with no warm-up or cool-down. Snow-shovelling is the classic scenario. Trouble strikes the avid hockey fan who leaps from the couch during the commercial break and attempts to shovel a foot of snow off the entire driveway before play resumes. But for those of us who make exercise a habit, the risk of heart trouble during exercise is very low. What's more, exercise significantly reduces the risk of dying suddenly from a heart attack during the twenty-four hours that follow a workout. Permanent bench warmers don't enjoy that benefit."

"How do you know when exercise is too much?" she asked.

"Keep the exercise intensity in the moderate range," I answered. "You should still be able to speak during the activity. Breathless panting means you've entered the high-intensity range. Heart rate is also a helpful guide. Here's a heart-rate range that you can target in the gym, based on today's testing." I handed Peter my exercise prescription. "That is, if you decide to break a sweat between now and next year's stress test."

Sample Exercise Prescription*

1. Warm-up
- Walk for 3–5 minutes at easy talking pace to warm leg muscles
- Warm-up target heart rate zone = 50–70% of maximum heart rate

2. Walk with intention at exercise pace for 30 minutes
- Break a sweat but still be able to talk
- Target heart rate zone = 70–85% of maximum heart rate, but 50–70% is okay if breaking a sweat is new territory for you and you need some time to get better conditioned
- Option of interspersing 1–2 minutes of easy walking every 10 minutes until conditioned

3. Cool down
- Walk easily for 3–5 minutes at comfortable talking pace again, to cool down
- After you stop, heart rate should drop by > 12

bpm after first minute of rest and > 22 bpm after two minutes of rest

4. Stretch

- Hamstring stretch: standing a metre from wall, lean forward, placing outstretched hands at shoulder width on wall as if being frisked by police, feeling gentle stretch in calves
- Quadriceps stretch: using a wall for balance, bend one leg at the knee, and holding onto ankle, pull heel up to buttocks for a gentle stretch of the thigh muscles
- Repeat sequence 3 to 6 times per week
- Alternatives to walking include elliptical trainer, stair climber, cycling, swimming, rowing

* Never begin an exercise program without consulting your doctor.

8

SUBTRACTING ADDICTION

A New Hope

"Which Star Wars movie do you like best?" my five-year-old asked as part of his bedtime stalling technique.

"The first one, of course," I answered without hesitation, remembering back to when the landmark film hit the theatres in 1977. (I saw it three times, paying for it with money I'd saved from my paper route.)

"You mean *Episode IV: A New Hope*," he corrected. Then he went on to ask, "*Why* do you like that one, Daddy? There's no cool fighting in it."

Wanting to defend Alec Guinness for a job well done, I lobbed back, "Because back then the writers could write and the actors could act! And besides, that final scene when the rebel forces attack the Death Star — that was pretty cool!"

"Yeah, I guess. But I still think Jar Jar Binks is better," he said, then yawned and dozed off.

George Lucas has been helpful in my clinic; I sometimes refer to this final scene from *Star Wars: Episode IV* to help illustrate some smoking-cessation issues with my patients. Stay with me. It's a brilliant analogy, and it may prove useful for you as well. It goes like this: You're Princess Leia. Well, I mean, she, the princess, represents all those who have been addicted to cigarette smoking, trapped in the clutches of nicotine's dark side, awaiting imminent execution. Darth Vader and his Nazi-like henchmen are the tobacco companies, thriving on deception and spreading death, destruction, and financial strain. And the remnant rebel forces — who courageously take on the giant forces of evil against all odds, in a valiant attempt to restore peace and harmony to the known universe — they're the medical profession, including, of course, yours truly (typecasting has its advantages).

Trapped in Addiction

"Sure, I tried smoking once," I readily confessed to Peter when he asked me about it in a defensive tone. "It was quite a while ago. I was at a drive-in movie theatre, watching *The Rocky Horror Picture Show*. There were six of us teens packed into an old Buick, and I made the mistake of sitting in the middle of the back seat. When we all lit up, the car was instantly transformed into a gas chamber. By the time I could scramble out to catch a breath, I was overcome with a fit of coughing and I threw up an allowance's worth of popcorn on the grass. I vowed never to smoke again."

"You're lucky," Peter said. "I wish I would've wimped out like that, too, instead of getting stuck smoking most of my life."

Hmm, I thought to myself. He seems to be softening up a tad. So I decided to launch into my best Columbo impersonation, complete with squinty eyes and hand gesturing (but no cigar). "So help me out here, Peter. With everything we know about smoking — how it causes heart disease, stroke, lung cancer, and all — what is it that you like about puffing your life away?"

"Not much really," he admitted. "It's just a bad habit."

Is smoking bad? Yes, most certainly. *A habit?* For the vast majority of those that smoke, yes again. But is smoking *just* a bad habit? No, I think not. Bad habits are like not wiping your feet on the entrance mat, not washing your hands before dinner, or picking your nose in public. Smoking is not just a bad habit — it's much more; otherwise, with a little bit of Dr. Skinner's behavioural modification, we'd have it licked. No, it's more than a habit. Smoking cigarettes is an *addiction.* More specifically, inhaling the nicotine in the cigarette is the addiction. Would anyone in their right mind want to huddle outside in the middle of winter to smoke a rolled-up tube of paper with dried leaves in it? Fat chance. But to calm the "nic-fit" storm, people will do just about anything. I witness this when I walk from my office to the hospital across the street; I see gowned patients pushing their IV poles down the snow-covered sidewalk in biting -20°C January air, bowing to the demands of their nicotine addiction.

Recognizing that the cigarette is merely the packaging container for the smoker's nicotine supply, one company got the idea of designing an e-cigarette — an *electronic* version of a cigarette. They eliminated everything in the cigarette, except for the nicotine. It's quite an ingenious little gadget: the electronic cigarette is a plastic rod that looks similar to a cigarette in size and shape. It has a replaceable cartridge filled with liquid nicotine that fits into the mouthpiece where you inhale, just like a regular cancer stick. The ingenious part is that there's a built-in microprocessor that detects air flow. So, when the "smoker" inhales through the tube, nicotine is injected in vapour form into the flowing air and to the lungs for absorption. To create that Casablanca ambience, the design team also added propylene glycol to the mix, which looks like smoke when vapourized, and gives the e-smoker that Humphrey Bogart appearance, with smoke rings rising. And if that's not enough, there's an orange LED at the tip of the tube that lights up to simulate a combusting cigarette. Not cheap, I'm sure, but it certainly makes the point that it's the nicotine, and nothing else, that is the cigarette's front-and-centre attraction.

Nicotine's name has a colourful bit of etymology. Similar to how we got Dentyne from combining the words *dental* plus *hygiene*, nicotine is also a word combo of sorts. The first part of nicotine, *nicot*, is named after the French Ambassador to Portugal back in the mid 1500s, Jean Nicot. The suffix *ine* generally refers to a chemical substance but, in this case, I wonder if the wordsmiths were thinking about *guillotine*. Ambassador Nicot is remembered, in part, for his political matchmaking role. He was given the task of negotiating a marriage between a six-year-old French princess and the five-year-old reigning king of Portugal, who, as it was said, "preferred older women." Although the kiddy prenuptials didn't prove successful, Nicot made the most of his foreign service by turning his attention to more adult activities, which included sampling the imported tobacco. Impressed by its medicinal potential (not!), he sent a collection of tobacco plants and seeds from Brazil to France for general consumption. He is credited with introducing snuff to the snooty French court, where it was initially frowned upon. But once the queen mother got hooked, everyone who was anyone in Paris was using tobacco in one form or another, spreading it throughout the west like the plague (… just like the Plague).

Also known as 1-methyl-2-(3-pyridyl) pyrolidine, nicotine is an oily extract found in tobacco leaves at a concentration less than 5 percent. This is a good thing, since in its pure form nicotine is highly poisonous — only one drop (50 mg) is fatal within minutes. But even in the lower concentration found in cigarette tobacco, nicotine negatively affects our cardiovascular system. It acts as a stimulant, increasing heart rate and blood pressure, and it adds to the vascular dysfunction seen in smokers. But these effects are relatively minor and certainly cannot account for the staggering death and destruction that smoking leaves in its wake. Nicotine attracts, but it doesn't kill. Like a bug light on the back porch, nicotine draws victims to danger, but doesn't do the actual zapping; that part is taken care of by the estimated 4,000 other chemicals and toxins found in cigarette smoke.[1] Front runners include carbon monoxide (generated by the incomplete combustion of tobacco, it impairs the ability of the blood to transport oxygen), tar, formaldehyde, hydrogen cyanide, and benzene. These toxins eventually kill, but the nicotine is the curse that keeps smokers coming back for more. Nicotine is one of the most addictive drugs known to mankind. That means that its right up there sharing the addiction spot light with the likes of heroin, cocaine, and even crack. Similar to dark chocolate with smooth caramel centres, it takes very little nicotine to engender a craving for more. After as few as two cigarettes, nicotine exposure changes the brain's neurochemistry enough to create chemical dependence.

How Deep Is Your Love for Cigarettes

Tobacco ads would have us believe that it's the taste of their particular brand of cigarette that attracts, but the truth is far less enticing and far more devious. It's all about the blood level of nicotine. Because nicotine is not a natural part of the body's chemistry, it is constantly removed from our circulation by the liver and destroyed. The dropping nicotine levels from your last cigarette trigger your desire for the next. This way, it's always the last cigarette you smoked that keeps you addicted. Why does the average smoker consume about fifteen to twenty cigarettes per day? Many smokers light up at least once every hour because they're trying to maintain their nicotine blood levels, whether they're aware of this or not. If nicotine is kept at a near constant level in the blood, then the veneer of contentedness is maintained. The tobacco industry knows that brand loyalty depends on how much nicotine smokers can get into their circulatory system and how fast; the more nicotine absorbed by the smoker, the bigger the nicotine rush, and the more devoted the addict.[2] To make cigarettes more addicting, there have been systematic increases in the nicotine yield from cigarettes sold in North America in recent years.[3] From 1998 to 2004, nicotine levels have increased by 10 percent, including those branded as "light." These efforts are solely to get smokers addicted more quickly and stay addicted longer.

In the brain, nicotine binds onto specific sites called the alpha4-beta2 receptors. Once activated, these receptors release neurotransmitters like dopamine into circulation, which then go on to activate our reward pathway and give us a sense of satisfaction. Eating, running, and lovemaking are other examples of behaviours that trigger this happy pathway (although, not necessarily in that order). Studies in neuroscience have shown that changes in neurotransmitter levels can result in actual architectural changes in the brain.[4] In other words, smoking can remodel the mind. It's been well studied in animals as well. Animal experiments show that mice and gorillas also develop withdrawal after nicotine exposure (mind you, many of the mice claimed they didn't inhale).

To help keep things even (the body is always trying to work towards balance or homeostasis), the numbers of nicotine receptors that smokers have are reduced over time. This means that to get the same nicotine effect you have to have more dopamine released by smoking more cigarettes. The medical community calls this phenomenon *tolerance*. The tobacco companies call it *record profits*. It is this increased requirement for dopamine to maintain the same electrical activity that is the basis of both physiological tolerance and withdrawal symptoms associated with nicotine addiction. So, by exploiting the brain's reward pathway, nicotine addiction produces a chronic relapsing brain disease. And like the treatment of any chronic illness, successful smoking cessation requires a long-term approach over a realistic timeline, optimized by professional assistance.

Not everyone suffers from the same degree of addiction to nicotine. The factors that govern the degree of addiction, or dependence, are complex and include the genetic predisposition (known as the addictive personality), the amount of exposure one has had to the drug (in this case, nicotine), and the time interval between the behaviour (smoking) and effect (nicotine on the brain). This instant gratification component is powerfully illustrated in cigarette smoking. It takes only about seven seconds for nicotine to hit the brain after a single drag; smoking is definitely the most efficient nicotine delivery system known to mankind. The lungs have such a large surface area (estimated at 70 m², or the size of a tennis court), that inhaled nicotine is instantaneously absorbed into the bloodstream faster than you can say, "I should really start cutting down how much I smoke."

One method to determine your level of nicotine dependence is by completing the Fagerstrom test.[7] This addiction tool makes use of a scoring system that stratifies nicotine dependence into mild (three points or less), moderate (four to six points) and severe (seven or more points). Generally, the more addicted you are, the more difficult it is to quit, and the more likely assistance will be needed to get the quit-for-life job done. Unfortunately, many smokers are so severely addicted that they make the till-death-do-us-part bond with the cigarette, and never successfully quit.

The Fagerstrom Test

1. How soon after you wake up do you smoke your first cigarette?
   a. Within 5 minutes — 3 points
   b. Between 6 and 30 minutes — 2 points
   c. Between 30 and 60 minutes — 1 point
   d. After 60 minutes — 0 points

2. Do you find it difficult to refrain from smoking in places where it is forbidden, such as in church, at the library, in the movie theatre?
   a. Yes — 1 point
   b. No — 0 points

3. Which cigarette would be the most difficult to give up?
   a. The first one in the morning — 1 point
   b. Any other cigarette — 0 points

4. How many cigarettes do you smoke in a day?
   a. Fewer than 10 — 0 points
   b. Between 10 and 20 — 1 point
   c. Between 20 and 30 — 2 points
   d. Over 30 — 3 points

5. Do you smoke more during the first few hours after waking than during the rest of the day?
   a. Yes — 1 point
   b. No — 0 points

6. Do you smoke even when you are so ill that you are in bed most of the time?
   a. Yes — 1 point
   b. No — 0 points

Results:
1–3 points = Mild dependence
4–6 points = Moderate dependence
7–10 points = Severe dependence

Source: Fagerstrom Test for Nicotine Dependence adapted with permission from T.F. Heatherton, et al., "The Fagerstrom Test for Nicotine Dependence: A Revision of the Fagerstrom Tolerance Questionnaire." *British Journal of Addictions* 86 (1991): 1119–27.

Excuses, and More Excuses

"No, Doc, you've got it all wrong," Peter said. "If you'd gotten onto smoking properly, you'd know that there's a lot more to it than just the nicotine rush. There are lots of reasons why people like to smoke."

Maybe he has a point; after all, I never did finish that first cigarette. I suppose one could argue that, as beauty is in the eye of the beholder, so cigarette enjoyment is in the mouth of the holder. But there's no getting around the highly addictive nicotine that tops the why-people-really-smoke charts. So, while the reasons abound as to why people may *think* they smoke, the reality of nicotine addiction remains. And where there's an addiction, rationalizations will rule the roost. Here are some common excuses about smoking that I'm frequently handed in my clinic.

It calms my nerves and helps me relax.

When non-smokers take a drag on a cigarette, they may experience a parched mouth, raunchy breath, and nausea, but they won't be calmed or relaxed. That's because non-smokers aren't addicted to nicotine — they don't crave nicotine, so smoking a cigarette holds no value. Nicotine is a stimulant. The stress hormone cortisol is measurably higher in those who smoke, supporting the observation that smokers are actually more anxious than the folks who don't. Those who smoke not only have life's issues coming at them, as everyone else does — mortgage payments, swamped social calendars, Christmas bills, photo radar speeding tickets, teenage body piercing — but they also have the unrelenting pangs throughout their waking hours to quench their nicotine addiction. To add insult to injury, smokers need to find a place where they're still allowed to light up. Our society has become hostile to the smoker. Today's outcast — the smoker — has become marginalized from mainstream events, institutions, and public transportation, and is forced to sneak into back alleys to top up blood nicotine levels. And if that's not enough to take away all tranquility, how about the financial strain of smoking? Pack-a-day smokers have to cough up over $3,000 of post-tax annual income to support their addiction. So much for calm and relaxation. No, the only stress relief that comes with smoking is the temporary respite from the nicotine withdrawal symptoms. And in an hour or so, as the blood nicotine level falls again, the nagging nicotine monster will be back.

I smoke because it clears my mind and helps me focus.

Smoking a cigarette may seem to be a more effective concentration aid than some other remedies, like Gotu Cola pills for example, but it's a misconception that smoking is helpful. Smoking a cigarette does nothing to improve brain function. Do neurosurgeons, facing a difficult case, scrub out for a smoke to rethink their surgical approach? Do commercial airline pilots light up when they hear of an approaching storm, so they can bring their wits to bear on negotiating the potential turbulence? Operating theatres and cockpits are arenas of intense and critical thinking, yet are smoke-free and by no coincidence. Granted, to fully concentrate, it's important to remove all distractions that could clutter your thoughts, and if you have nicotine cravings on your mind, smoking a cigarette may allow you to focus better. But that's only because the nicotine need is temporarily silenced. It's a bit like hitting your head against a wall; sure, it feels better when you stop, but that's hardly reason to do the damage in the first place. Those of us who are engaged in tasks that require a high level of concentration do not smoke.

I smoke to occupy myself. It's the way I deal with boredom.

When I think of mind-expanding activities, lighting a cigarette and puffing on it doesn't come to mind. So you want to fire a few neurons while you wait for the bus? How about a crossword or Sudoku puzzle, knitting a scarf for the mothers' shelter, or, better yet, penning out a letter to your mom (who probably hasn't heard from you in over six months)? Smoking is an anemic way of breaking monotony and only confirms boredom. If anything, smoking probably increases the chances of becoming bored; it offers an easy, mind-numbing activity for people who might otherwise have the energy, extra money, and motivation to seek genuine solutions to boredom. Many exciting activities, such as sports, are incompatible with smoking. Life is exciting. Being dead is boring. You choose.

I smoke to help control my weight. I'd gain twenty pounds if I quit.

Smoking is an ineffective and unhealthy weight-control method. And since the craving for cigarettes and the hunger for food are similar sensations, nicotine addiction renders smokers continuously hungry and liable to eat to quench the pangs of dependence. Thus, smoking may actually foster unhealthy weight gain.

Sure, nicotine can affect metabolism. Smoking a cigarette burns approximately ten calories.[5] So for a pack of coffin nails, that's about 200 calories and, for a pack-a-day smoker, puffing at it for two and a half weeks, it works out to about 3,500 calories, or one pound of flesh. "Not bad," you say? Well, Shylock may be happy, but your cardiovascular system isn't. If you had quit smoking for those two and a half weeks, your body would have enjoyed significant health gains, including improved uptake of oxygen by your lungs and muscles, reduced blood pressure, enhanced vascular function, significant lung repair, and a measurable reduction in both heart attack and stroke risk.[6] Which is more important? Yes, excess weight is hard on our health — abdominal obesity in particular. However, some of the weight gain that occurs after stopping smoking may be from healthy rehydration in the form of body water — not a bad thing. But whatever the cause, the potential weight gain related to smoking cessation is small peanuts by comparison to the health benefits that are derived from quitting. There are better ways to achieve weight control than by killing yourself.

I smoke for the pleasure of it. I like the taste.

To which I respond, "You *like* that yucky taste? What, are you eating the cigarettes and then licking the ash tray? Argh!" (Excuse me, I just had a flashback to my suffocating drive-in movie experience.) Let's be honest here. Smoking *doesn't* taste good. It's gross! Smokers smoke *despite* the bad taste. And more than just tasting awful, smoking damages our taste buds and the mucosal lining of our nasal passages, and reduces our ability to appreciate things that *do* taste good. Many reformed smokers confess to a realization of how good food actually tastes, once they've stopped smoking. No, there's no subtle fragrance, no spicy tropical undertones, no flutters of cherry, no delicate honey-nut finish, or any other refined taste experience that sucking on a smouldering cigarette can offer. The only pleasure that smoking provides is the transient relief of nicotine cravings. Real pleasure starts when you quit smoking, and the slavery to nicotine has ended.

Smoking is macho. It makes me feel cool.

If smoking icon James Dean hadn't been killed on the highway in his twenties and was given the opportunity to smoke into midlife, chances are his appeal would have soon faded. Joining the ranks of other long-term smokers, like Dean Martin, he also would have become prematurely wizened, grey-skinned, and impotent, saddled with a chronic, hacking cough, and most probably even tethered to on oxygen cylinder to breathe — goodbye macho sex symbol, hello train wreck.

An American study found a link between towns with tough controls to keep kids from buying cigarettes and lower crime rates. Those towns that aggressively enforced youth tobacco laws had the lowest rates of crime, including violent and property crime.[8] Not that smoking causes such behaviour, but it may very well foster the rebels-without-a-cause attitude. As unfortunate as it is, it's understandable that teens chase after the cool image of pouty lips dangling a cigarette, since their whole world is being rocked with hormones and hang-ups. What they see advertised on billboards or in the movie theatres speaks to their insecurities. But the upside-down world of adolescence, where appearance is everything, should end with the high school twenty-year reunion — the smokers didn't age well in my class. We all need to acknowledge that it's what's on the inside that's important, and inside a smoker are black lungs and narrowed blood vessels. "Nothing *cool* here folks, just move right along now."

The sun-cured hint of sweetness taste, the improved concentration capacity, the pillow-soft relaxation opportunities, and the outdoor adventurer persona have nothing to do with smoking cigarettes and everything to do with cleverly crafted lies, perpetuated by the tobacco industry. These falsehoods have paid the tobacco companies dividends in the order of billions of dollars annually from nicotine-addicted Canadians, many of whom are children. Their primary goal is selling their product — a product that kills those who take it as directed.

The Tobacco Empire Strikes Back

Over the past twenty years, significant inroads have been made on the anti-smoking front. A combination of massive public health campaigns, use of warning labels on cigarette packages, no-smoking laws that limit public smoking opportunities, stringent tobacco

Subtracting Addiction

marketing regulations, and escalating cigarette taxation have all contributed to the declining smoking rates in high-income countries, like Canada. But the tobacco giants haven't taken this lying down and have tried their best to keep pace. The tobacco industry has marketed its cigarettes using a wide array of product varieties with catchy adjectives and slogans to give the purchaser the delusion of choice: you've got your wides, regulars, slims, 100s, 120s, unfiltered, full filter, lights, ultra lights, menthol, house blends. They're all just minor variations on the same, deadly theme. It's all about providing nicotine to hook you and keep you hooked. To disguise their real intentions, and appear to satisfy the growing desire of smokers to reduce nicotine and tar levels, tobacco companies have dreamed up cigarette ventilation systems, supposedly designed to reduce noxious fume inhalation. But they don't work. Unfortunately, half of the tiny ventilation holes get blocked by the users' lips or hands and don't make a great deal of difference in reducing smoke fumes inhaled. As well, it's been clearly shown that a smoker will drag on a cigarette until the desired nicotine level has been reached. So, regardless of the labelled nicotine content, or the presence of ventilation holes, smokers inhale until they get what they want. If there's less nicotine in the cigarette, then there's more lung-busting inhaling. In an attempt to make their cigarettes appear more health friendly, companies underscore the branding of low tar or ultra light. But it's just more of the same snake-oil salesman marketing. There is no *safe* amount to smoke and no *healthy* brand to choose from. Court orders have been issued to stop tobacco companies from using such monikers, because they only serve to deceive the public about the perils of smoking.

This type of negative exposure has been bad for business. So to ensure survival in an increasingly hostile environment, the tobacco industry has been forced to find other markets on the globe to exploit. Who better to pick on than the developing countries and vulnerable populations? "Blessed are the meek," right? When I was in Kenya, I saw starter packs of three cigarettes held together by an elastic band being distributed to adults and children alike, at a nominal cost, in the hopes that addiction would get a foothold. It is predicted by the World Health Organization that within the next twenty years almost three-quarters of smoking-related deaths will be occurring in low and middle-income countries.[9]

In Canada, likewise, the northern communities have been heavily targeted by tobacco companies and offered cigarettes at reduced prices. This is compounded by the illicit tobacco trade that operates vigorously on reserves, with annual sales estimated in the hundreds of millions of dollars. As a result, nearly 60 percent of First Nations and Inuit people in Canada smoke, which is more than double the rate for the rest of the country. The teen situation is especially desperate. First Nations boys between the ages of fifteen and seventeen years have a smoking rate of nearly 50 percent, climbing to over 60 percent for girls of the same age range, and amounting to over four times the national average. To break your heart further, almost 60 percent of pregnant First Nations women smoke, passing on the harmful toxins to the next generation.[10] Someone is getting rich, while countless others are getting sick and dying.

China has become the latest tobacco marketing Mecca. Of the 1.3 billion smokers worldwide, China is home to a full one-third of the total.[11] This problem has been exacerbated by the involvement of the home government in the dirty deed, with tobacco sales generating nearly 8 percent of China's total revenue. Current marketing strategies are aimed at China's children, with the use of candy-flavoured cigarettes — not the Popeye varieties, either. As well, East Asian teens and so-called liberated women are enticed by imported images of Western independence, and thrilled to be told that "you've come a long way baby." Despite the reports from Asian researchers showing that the risk of lung cancer can drop by 70 percent if smoking is stopped, massive numbers embrace the bad habit. As a result, heart disease and cancer rates in Asia are forecasted to climb exponentially.

Smoking only pays dividends to big business, and impoverishes everyone else who is within range of the odour. For too long, the tobacco industry has successfully marketed smoking as exciting and glamorous, disguising the tragedy of addiction behind facades of adventure, freedom, success, and beauty. Smoking promises much,

Subtracting Addiction

but delivers only dirty drapes and premature death certificates. At the end of the day, we're like the onlookers in Hans Christian Anderson's "The Emperor's New Clothes." The pleasures of smoking are lies that have been painstakingly woven into the fabric of our society, to the point where many believe them to be true. Far worse than simply being left empty-handed (or in the case of the naked king, embarrassed), smoking cigarettes leaves us financially drained and at risk for serious health problems.

Targeting the Death Star

Let's get back to that *Star Wars: Episode IV* analogy. As you recall, seconds before her capture, Princess Leia was able to download the secret technical plans of the Death Star into her little droid, R2D2, and send him for help. At the story's end, just as the Empire's planet-like super weapon is jockeying for position to make toast of the rebel alliance, the Death Star's blueprints are reviewed and a weakness is discovered. Enter Cool Hand Luke, who exploits the weakness and saves the day. Now for the analogy: the biology of nicotine addiction has also been studied in detail. And like the rebel alliance, the medical community has found a number of weak points that can be exploited to aid those wishing to quit smoking.

The Nicotine Target

Fighting fire with fire may sound like trading one problem for another, but using nicotine replacement therapy (NRT) has been shown to double the odds of successful quitting.[12] Many fear nicotine and, although nicotine isn't devoid of problems for the cardiovascular system, these effects are quite minor by comparison to what's caused by the 4,000-some-odd chemicals found in cigarette smoke. The beauty of NRT is that it helps to separate the behaviour of smoking from the nicotine addiction. Nicotine replacement allows you to tackle the habit part of smoking, and later, slowly wean off the addictive nicotine. To boost the success rates further, NRT can be used with other smoking cessation aids, under the direction of an MD.

There are a fair number of nicotine-replacement therapies to choose from (see the bulleted list on the next page) and, since they're considered over-the-counter medications, you don't need a doctor's prescription. They're all equally effective; the choice of replacement is one of personal preference. Although NRT supplies nicotine to the body, it doesn't increase blood levels as instantaneously as smoking, but gets absorbed more slowly, deconditioning the instant-gratification connection.

Side effects to NRT formulations are not usually an issue, occurring in less than 5 percent of users. NRT isn't recommended in pregnancy, since nicotine can cause low birth weight, and the effects on the developing fetal brain are unknown. As well, NRT isn't recommended in the days following a heart attack or stroke (although we occasionally make an exception to this rule, since many physicians feel that either ongoing smoking or untreated nicotine withdrawal is more of a risk than the replacement drug).[13] Lastly, since it is possible to overdose on nicotine, or become addicted to the heightened amounts, it's important not to smoke while using NRT.

The patch is a popular device for NRT. It allows nicotine to get slowly absorbed through the skin into the bloodstream. Since a single cigarette supplies about 1 milligram (mg) of nicotine to the blood, daily patch strength varies (7 mg, 14 mg, and 21 mg, strengths), so that users can mimic their usual nicotine exposure from smoking. For example, for those who smoke a pack or more a day (twenty or more cigarettes), the 21 mg patch will best approximate the desired blood levels. It's recommended that every two weeks, the patch strength be reduced. This allows you to slowly wean from the nicotine and minimize withdrawal symptoms.

Potential problems with nicotine patches include insomnia and vivid dreams (especially if it's worn at night).[14] Since the patch can cause some skin irritation, those with adhesive allergy (like me) should avoid them. To minimize mild skin reactions, it's recommended to change placement sites now and again — but don't forget to take the patch off at day's end. I had one elderly patient who had six patches plastered over various parts of his body (which he had completely forgotten about). "Well, no wonder I was feeling a bit shaky," he remarked, as I helped him peel off the excess patches.

Nicotine gum is also a popular choice, perhaps because of the oral stimulation and the opportunity to expend nervous energy. The slow-release design of the gum works best if you park it in between the teeth and the cheek, rather than chewing it. Side effects include a tingling sensation in the mouth, hiccups, nausea, heartburn, and, of course, the terrible taste (I learned this the hard way when my brother-in-law secretly traded my Dentyne for a stick of Nicorette gum — yikes!). But despite the acquired taste, many former smokers continue to happily chew nicotine replacement gum for years, with little, if any, medical concerns. Some of my patients use gum combined with the patch for extra effect.

The nicotine inhaler is like a poor man's version of the e-cigarette. It works like an asthmatic's puffer and effectively delivers nicotine in vapour form to the mouth and throat. Many prefer it because it simulates the hand-to-mouth behaviour of smoking, without the smoking. Inhaler side effects include cough, a scratchy throat sensation, and nausea. It's not recommended for asthmatics, but then again, neither is smoking.

Delivery System

- patch
- gum
- inhaler
- nasal spray
- lozenge
- slow-release tablet

Target the Receptor

Drugs that can bind onto the nicotine receptors in the brain can be used to short-circuit the effects of the drug. A relatively new kid on the pharmaceutical block, varenicline (Champix in Canada or Chantix in the United States) was designed to help reduce both the cravings of nicotine and some of the so-called pleasurable effects of nicotine.[15] This Yin-Yang pill accomplishes these seemingly opposite effects by turning on the nicotine receptor, but only halfway. It's called a partial agonist, and is comparable to getting to second base (in high school dating jargon). The beauty of this approach is that it occupies the receptor so that nicotine isn't needed, but it doesn't provide the associated nicotine rush. As a result, nicotine from a smoked cigarette becomes redundant. Whatever enjoyment there was from the cigarette quickly fades away and becomes a distant memory. So, it's easier to give the next cigarette a miss, and in time, ditch them all together.

Varenicline is taken twice a day for twelve weeks, during which time patients are encouraged to choose a quit date. It's not recommended for those under eighteen, since it was tested only on adults. Likewise, no sane pharmaceutical company would miss the usual disclaimer "not to be used in pregnancy or while lactating," since who knows how any drug may affect the developing babe. Side effects of varenicline include headache, insomnia or abnormal dreams, altered taste sensation, nausea (which can be quite disabling), vomiting (quite messy), and flatulence (better out than in).

The unfortunate death of musician Carter Albrecht raised concerns about possible psychological side effects of the drug. Although he was taking Varenicline at the time he was tragically shot to death, reports say that his blood alcohol level was three times the legal driving limit. So, his untimely death likely had more to do with gun legislation issues and alcohol excess, than with side effects from taking the smoking cessation aid. Nonetheless, Canadian Varenicline labels warn of an increased risk of suicidal behaviour, depression, and agitation.

Subtracting Addiction

Target the Brain

Buproprion (Wellbutrin or Zyban) is a neurotransmitter stabilizer that helps counteract the effects of nicotine on the brain.[16] Specifically, the drug blocks the re-uptake of dopamine, so it ends up hanging around longer, stabilizing mood and reducing the urge to light up. The drug was initially used as an antidepressant, and, during its debut, it was noted that patients taking buproprion were able to quit smoking more easily.[17] Buproprion showed a double benefit: good-bye dreary blues and hello fresh blue sky. As with the nicotine replacement options, research suggests that the chances of successfully quitting double with buproprion on the ship deck — permission to come aboard the *Love Boat*, Captain Stubing. And the odds are even better when used together with nicotine replacement therapy.

Potential side effects of buproprion include dry mouth, nausea, insomnia, tremor, increase in sweating, ringing in the ears, and skin rash. But, hey, no pain, no gain. As well, similar to most anti-depressants, it lowers the seizure threshold. That means that if someone is predisposed to having seizures, this medication is a bad choice. This was the reason Wellbutrin was initially removed from the market — seizure city. But after a dose reduction and the cautionary note that it shouldn't be used by those with mood disorders, eating disorders, or epilepsy, all has been reasonably quiet on the litigation front.

As helpful as buproprion and other cessation aids may be, successful quitting still requires willpower and is made easier with some intentional planning. Setting a quit date to get the mind on board significantly improves the effectiveness of any of the chosen medication aids. Even little things like removing cigarettes from the car and making the house a smoke-free zone as the date approaches increases success rates substantially.

Any Last Words?

Peter was seated quietly in front of the window when I walked into the exercise lab.

"That time of the year so soon?" I asked.

He nodded. "You say the same thing every year."

"Yes, I like to be consistent. But doesn't it just seem like yesterday since you were here last?" As Peter stepped up onto the treadmill, I said, "Here's a line of questioning that I guess I also repeat ad nauseam. 'How's the smoking going now? Have you been able to cut down any since last year's assessment?'"

"Quit," he said in a deliberately understated tone as a smile slowly spread across his whiskered face.

"You what?" I squealed. "How? I mean, what happened? Well, that's wonderful. Did you get help? Was it hard? You … you quit!" I stammered in staccato succession, thunderstruck by the good news.

"Naw, I just went cold turkey. I got tired of all the fuss, pitched my pack in the wastepaper basket, and got on with things."

Trying to recompose myself, I held out my hand to congratulate him. "You've just made my day, Peter. I'm so happy for you. Welcome to the first day of the rest of your life!"

Cold turkey is certainly an option. Many of my patients who have suffered a heart attack give up smoking all at once, and do so successfully. It seems that a near-death experience can be quite the motivation for change. But regardless of the cessation mode, there is no better time to quit than right this instant. If you're serious about improving heart health, you have to stop smoking. This is an iron-clad fact that cannot be avoided. Of course, you don't have to face the challenge alone. Your family doctor, dietician, personal trainer, and friends who have successfully quit smoking are some important examples of people who can help see you through to improved heart health, smoke-free forever.

Although I've shared some ideas about how vascular injury might be mitigated in the face of smoking exposure, these beneficial factors pale by comparison to the benefits afforded by smoking cessation itself. Every single mechanism of vascular injury outlined with the PLAC diagram, from the platelet activation and vascular lining injury, to blood vessel wall inflammation and cholesterol core buildup, is made worse by smoking (see Figure 8.1). So much so, that it would be irresponsible to suggest that smokers can achieve acceptable heart health while continuing to smoke. In time, everyone will stop smoking. The trick is to maximize the time interval between your last cigarette and your last breath. If Peter can do it, you can, too!

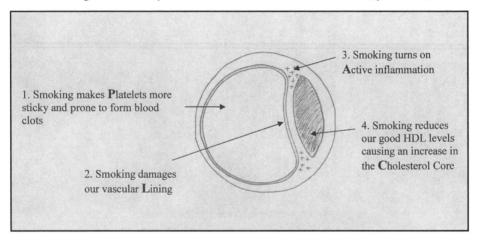

1. Smoking makes **P**latelets more sticky and prone to form blood clots

2. Smoking damages our vascular **L**ining

3. Smoking turns on **A**ctive inflammation

4. Smoking reduces our good HDL levels causing an increase in the **C**holesterol Core

Figure 8.1: PLAC summary for the harmful effects of smoking.

NOTES

Foreword

1. J.O. Prochaska and C.C. DiClemente, "Stages of Change in the Modification of Problem Behaviors." *Progress in Behavior Modification* 28 (1992): 183–218. Review article.

Introduction

1. N. Kohler and B. Righton, *Maclean's*, April 18, 2006.

Chapter 1: Risky Business

1. *The Heart and Stroke Foundation* 2004 Canadian mortality data from Statistics Canada. www.heartandstroke.com/site/c. ikIQLcMWJtE/b.3483991/k.34A8/Statistics.htm#deaths (accessed November 13, 2008).

2. P.D. Thompson, "Historical Aspects of the Athlete's Heart." D. Bruce Dill Historical Lecture. *Medicine & Science in Sports & Exercise* 36(3) (2004): 363–70.

3. A. Kagan, et al., "The Framingham Study: A Prospective Study of Coronary Heart Disease." *Federation Proceedings* 21(4) Part 2 (July–August 1962): 52–57.

4. S. Yusuf, et al., INTERHEART Study Investigators. "Obesity and the Risk of Myocardial Infarction in 27,000 Participants from 52 Countries: A Case-Control Study." *Lancet* 366(9497) (November 5, 2005): 1640–49.

5. S.M. Grundy, et al., "Assessment of Cardiovascular Risk by Use of Multiple-Risk-Factor Assessment Equations: A Statement for Healthcare Professionals from the American Heart Association and the American College of Cardiology." *Circulation* 100(13) (September 28, 1999): 1481–92.

6. R. Kahn, et al., "The Impact of Prevention on Reducing the Burden of Cardiovascular Disease." *Circulation* (2008) July 7.

7. T.K. Fenske, "Preventing the Next Heart Attack." *Patient Care* 15(8) (August 2004): 44–53.

8. W.B. Kannel, et al., "An Investigation of Coronary Heart Disease in Families: The Framingham Offspring Study." *American Journal of Epidemiology* 110(3) (September 1979): 281–90.

9. R. Huxley, et al., "Waist Circumference Thresholds Provide an Accurate and Widely Applicable Method for the Discrimination of Diabetes." *Diabetes Care* 30(12) (December 2007): 3116–18.

10. S. Zhu, et al., "Waist Circumference and Obesity-Associated Risk Factors Among Whites in the Third National Health and Nutrition

Examination Survey: Clinical Action Thresholds." *American Journal of Clinical Nutrition* 76(4) (October 2002): 743–49.

Chapter 2: Blood Is Thicker Than Water

1. Physicians' Health Study Research Group. *New England Journal of Medicine*. 321(3) (July 20, 1989): 129–35.

2. A.T. Chan, et al., "Long-Term Aspirin Use and Mortality in Women." *Archives of Internal Medicine* 167(6) (March 26, 2007): 562–72.

3. Antiplatelet Trialists. "Collaborative Meta-Analysis of Randomised Trials of Antiplatelet Therapy for Prevention of Death, Myocardial Infarction, and Stroke in High Risk Patients." *British Medical Journal* 324(7329) (January 12, 2002): 71–86.

4. N. Rodondi, et al. Health, Aging, and Body Composition Study Research Group. "Aspirin Use for the Primary Prevention of Coronary Heart Disease in Older Adults." *American Journal of Medicine* 118(11) (November 2005): 1288.

5. J. Cui, et al., "What Do Commercial Ginseng Preparations Contain?" *Lancet* 344(8915) (July 9, 1994): 134.

6. A. Poli, et al. Nutrition Foundation of Italy. "Non-Pharmacological Control of Plasma Cholesterol Levels." *Nutrition, Metabolism & Cardiovascular Diseases* 18(2) (February 2008): S1–16.

7. R. McPherson, et al. Canadian Cardiovascular Society. "Canadian Cardiovascular Society Position Statement — Recommendations for the Diagnosis and Treatment of Dyslipidemia and Prevention of Cardiovascular Disease." *Canadian Journal of Cardiology* 22(11) (September 2006): 913–27.

Chapter 3: Defending the Lining

1. M.R. Joffres, et al., "Awareness, Treatment, and Control of Hypertension in Canada." *American Journal of Hypertension* 10(10 Part 1) (October 1997): 1097–1102.

2. N.R. Campbell, et al., "Canadian Hypertension Education Program Outcomes Research Task Force." *Canadian Journal of Cardiology* 24(6) (June 2008): 485–90.

3. V. Aram, et al., and the National High Blood Pressure Education Program Coordinating Committee, "The Seventh Report of the Joint National Committee on Prevention, Detection, Evaluation, and Treatment of High Blood Pressure." *Journal of the American Medical Association* 289(2003): (doi: 10.1001/ Journal of the American Medical Association.289.19.2560).

4. V. Franco, S. Oparil, and O.A. Carretero. "Hypertensive Therapy: Part I." *Circulation* 109(24) (June 22, 2004): 2953–58.

5. S. Havas, B. Dickinson, and M. Wilson, "The Urgent Need to Reduce Sodium Consumption." *Journal of the American Medical Association* 298 (2007): 1439–41.

6. L.J. Appel, et al. DASH Collaborative Research Group. "A Clinical Trial of the Effects of Dietary Patterns on Blood Pressure." *New England Journal of Medicine* 336(16) (April 17, 1997): 1117–24.

7. N.A. Khan, et al. Canadian Hypertension Education Program. "The 2008 Canadian Hypertension Education Program Recommendations for the Management of Hypertension: Part 2 — Therapy." *Canadian Journal of Cardiology* 24(6) (June 2008): 465–75.

Chapter 4: You Snooze or You Lose

1. J.R. Espiritu, "Age–Related Sleep Changes." *Clinics in Geriatric Medicine* 24(1) (February 2008): 1–14, v.

2. S. Jelic, et al., "Inflammation, Oxidative Stress, and Repair Capacity of the Vascular Endothelium in Obstructive Sleep Apnea." *Circulation* 117(17) (April 29, 2008): 2270–78.

3. G. Jean-Louis, et al., "Obstructive Sleep Apnea and Cardiovascular Disease: Role of the Metabolic Syndrome and Its Components." *Journal of Clinical Sleep Medicine* 4(3) (June 15, 2008): 261–72.

4. P. Dorasamy, "Obstructive Sleep Apnea and Cardiovascular Risk." *Journal of Therapeutics and Clinical Risk Managment* 3(6) (Dec 2007): 1105–11.

5. J.M. Lyznicki, et al., "Sleepiness, Driving, and Motor Vehicle Crashes." *Journal of the American Medical Association* 279 (1998): 1908–13.

6. A. Samel, M. Vejvoda, and H. Maass, "Sleep Deficit and Stress Hormones in Helicopter Pilots on 7-Day Duty for Emergency Medical Services." *Aviation, Space and Environmental Medicine* 75(11) (November 2004): 935–40.

7. J.M. Lyznicki, et al.

8. H. Moldofsky, et al., "Musculosketal Symptoms and Non–REM Sleep Disturbance in Patients with 'Fibrositis Syndrome' and Healthy Subjects." *Psychosomatic Medicine* 37(4) (July–August 1975): 341–51.

9. S. Jelic, et al., "Inflammation, Oxidative Stress, and Repair Capacity of the Vascular Endothelium in Obstructive Sleep

Apnea." *Circulation* 117(17) (April 29, 2008): 2270–78.

10. Pagel, J.F. "Medication Effects on Sleep." *Dental Clinics of North America* 45(4) (October 2001): 855–65.

11. N. Cimolai, "Zopiclone: Is It a Pharmacologic Agent for Abuse?" *Canadian Family Physician* 53(12) (December 2007): 2124–29.

12. M.W. Johns, "A New Method for Measuring Daytime Sleepiness: The Epworth Sleepiness Scale." *Sleep* 14 (6) (1991): 540–45.

Chapter 5: Tooth Fairy Confidential

1. K.K. Kwang, H.H. Seung, and M.J. Quon, "Inflammatory Markers and the Metabolic Syndrome: Insights from Therapeutic Interventions." *Journal of the American College of Cardiology* 46 (2005): 1978–85.

2. P.M. Ridker, et al., "Comparison of C-Reactive Protein and Low-Density Lipoprotein Cholesterol Levels in the Prediction of First Cardiovascular Events." *New England Journal of Medicine* 347(20) (November 14, 2002): 1557–65.

3. B. Zethelius, et al., "Use of Multiple Biomarkers to Improve the Prediction of Death from Cardiovascular Causes." *New England Journal of Medicine* 358(20) (May 15, 2008): 2107–16.

4. M.S. Tonetti, et al., "Treatment of Periodontitis and Endothelial Function." *New England Journal of Medicine* 356(9) (March 1, 2007): 911–20.

5. W.J. Millar and D. Locker, "Smoking and Oral Health." *Journal of the Canadian Dental Association* March 73(2) (2007): 155–55g.

6. C. Liena-Puy, "The Role of Saliva in Maintaining Oral Health and as an Aid to Diagnosis." *Medicina Oral, Patología Oral y Cirugía Bucal* 11(5) (August 2006): E449–55.

7. T.K. Fenske and D.A. Taylor, "Infective Endocarditis Reviewed." *Canadian Journal of Cardiology* 13 (1997): 329.

8. D.K. Lam, et al. American Heart Association. "Prevention of Infective Endocarditis: Revised Guidelines from the American Heart Association and the Implications for Dentists." *Journal of the Canadian Dental Association* 74(5) (June 2008): 449–53.

9. J.M. ten Cate, "Biofilms, a New Approach to the Microbiology of Dental Plaque." *Odontology* 94(1) (September 2006): 1–9.

10. A.F. Paes Leme, et al., "The Role of Sucrose in Cariogenic Dental Biofilm Formation — New Insight." *Journal of Dental Research* 85(10) (October 2006): 878–87.

11. G.K. Johnson and M. Hill, "Cigarette Smoking and the Periodontal Patient." *Journal of Periodontology* 75(2) (February 2004): 196–209.

12. G. Holm, "Smoking as an Additional Risk for Tooth Loss." *Journal of Periodontology* 65(11) (November 1994): 996–1001.

13. C.W. Douglass, "Risk Assessment and Management of Periodontal Disease." *Journal of the American Dental Association* 137(supplement 3) (2006): 27S–32S.

14. S.L. Tomar and S. Asma, "Smoking-Attributable Periodontitis in the United States: Findings from NHANES III. National Health and Nutrition Examination Survey." *Journal of Periodontology* 71(5) (May 2000): 743–51.

15. B.A. Matis, et al., "Extended Bleaching of Tetracycline-Stained Teeth: A 5-Year Study." *Operative Dentistry* 31(6) (November–December 2006): 643–51.

16. L.E. Tam, V.Y. Kuo, and A. Norooz, "Effect of Prolonged Direct and Indirect Peroxide Bleaching on Fracture Toughness of Human Dentin." *Journal of Esthetic and Restorative Dentistry* 19(2) (2007): 100–09.

17. M.L. Barnett, "The Rationale for the Daily Use of an Antimicrobial Mouthrinse." *Journal of the American Dental Association* 137(supplement 3) (November 2006): 16S–21S.

18. J. Kolahi and A. Soolari, "Rinsing with Chlorhexidine Gluconate Solution After Brushing and Flossing Teeth: A Systematic Review of Effectiveness." *Quintessence International* 37(8) (September 2006): 605–12.

19. R.E. Horseman, "Open Wide: Here Comes IntelliDrug." *Journal of the California Dental Association* 35(6) (June 2007): 453–54.

Chapter 6: Gut Reaction

1. G.L. Burke, et al., "The Impact of Obesity on Cardiovascular Disease Risk Factors and Subclinical Vascular Disease: The Multi-Ethnic Study of Atherosclerosis." *Archives of Internal Medicine* 168(9) (May 12, 2008): 928–35.

2. R.H. Eckel, "Clinical Practice: Nonsurgical Management of Obesity in Adults." *New England Journal of Medicine* 358 (2008): 1941–50.

3. D.C. Lau, et al. Obesity Canada Clinical Practice Guidelines Expert Panel. "2006 Canadian Clinical Practice Guidelines

on the Management and Prevention of Obesity in Adults and Children [Summary]." *Journal of the Canadian Medical Association* 176(8) (April 10, 2007): S1–13. Review.

4. J.P. Després, et al., "Abdominal Obesity and the Metabolic Syndrome: Contribution to Global Cardiometabolic Risk." *Arteriosclerosis, Thrombosis, and Vascular Biology* 28(6) (June 2008): 1039–49.

5. P.L. Lutsey, L.M. Steffen, and J. Stevens, "Dietary Intake and the Development of the Metabolic Syndrome: The Atherosclerosis Risk in Communities Study." *Circulation* 117(6) (February 12, 2008): 754–61.

6. A. Benetos, et al., "All-Cause and Cardiovascular Mortality Using the Different Definitions of Metabolic Syndrome." *American Journal of Cardiology* 102(2) (July 15, 2008): 188–91.

7. C.M. Ballantyne, et al., "Metabolic Syndrome Risk for Cardiovascular Disease and Diabetes in the ARIC Study." *International Journal of Obesity (London)* 32 Supplement 2 (May 2008): S21–24.

8. T.K. Fenske and M. Elhatton, "Dietary Advice for Your Post-MI Patient." *Patient Care* 12(6) (2001): 72–83.

Chapter 7: Core Curriculum

1. The Scandinavian Simvastatin Survival Study (4S). "Randomised Trial of Cholesterol Lowering in 4444 Patients with Coronary Heart Disease." *Lancet* 344(8934) (November 19, 1994): 1383–89.

2. T.K. Fenske, "CV Risk Assessment: So Many Options, So Little

Time." *Perspectives in Cardiology* 23(10) (November–December 2007): 27–30.

3. M. Coylewright, R.S. Blumenthal, and W. Post, "Placing COURAGE in Context: Review of the Recent Literature on Managing Stable Coronary Artery Disease." *Proceedings of the Mayo Clinic* 83(7) (July 2008): 799–805.

4. G.M. Sangiorgi, et al., "Plaque Vulnerability and Related Coronary Event Prediction by Intravascular Ultrasound with Virtual Histology: 'It's a Long Way to Tipperary'?" *Catheterizations and Cardiovascular Interventions* 70(2) (August 1, 2007): 203–10.

5. S. Glagov, E. Weisenberg, and C.K. Zarins. *New England Journal of Medicine* 316 (1987): 1371.

6. A.P. Schroeder and E. Falk, "Vulnerable and Dangerous Coronary Plaques." *Atherosclerosis* 118 Supplement (December 1995): S141–49.

7. H.B. Rubins, et al., "Gemfibrozil for the Secondary Prevention of Coronary Heart Disease in Men with Low Levels of High-Density Lipoprotein Cholesterol: Veterans Affairs High-Density Lipoprotein Cholesterol Intervention Trial Study Group." *New England Journal of Medicine* 341(6) (August 5, 1999): 410–18.

8. P.W. Wilson, "High-Density Lipoprotein, Low-Density Lipoprotein and Coronary Artery Disease." *American Journal of Cardiology* 66(6) (September 4, 1990): 7A–10A.

9. T.R. Joy and R.A. Hegele, "The Failure of Torcetrapib: What Have We Learned?" *British Journal of Pharmacology* (June 9, 2008): 1379–81.

10. M.H. Davidson and P.P. Toth, "High-Density Lipoprotein Metabolism: Potential Therapeutic Targets." *American Journal of Cardiology* 100(11 A) (December 3, 2007): n32–40.

11. D.W. de Lange, "From Red Wine to Polyphenols and Back: A Journey Through the History of the French Paradox." *Thrombosis Research* 119(4) (2007): 403–06. Epub July 12, 2006.

12. T.K. Fenske, "Alcohol and the Heart: A Look at Both Sides." *Perspectives in Cardiology* 24(5) (May 2008): 27–30.

13. J.H. O'Keefe, K.A. Bybee, and C.J. Lavie, "Alcohol and Cardiovascular Health: The Razor-Sharp Double-Edged Sword." *Journal of the American College of Cardiology* 50(11) (September 11, 2007): 1009–14.

14. E.R. Gritz, et al., "National Working Conference on Smoking and Body Weight. Task Force 3: Implications with Respect to Intervention and Prevention." *Health Psychology* 11 Supplement (1992): 17–25. Review.

15. A. Di Castelnuovo, et al., "Alcohol Dosing and Total Mortality in Men and Women: An Updated Meta-Analysis of 34 Prospective Studies." *Archives of Internal Medicine* 166(22) (December 11–25, 2006): 2437–45.

16. P.T. Katzmarzyk, N. Gledhill, and R.J. Shephard, "The Economic Burden of Physical Inactivity in Canada." *Journal of the Canadian Medical Association* 163(11) (November 28, 2000): 1435–40.

17. C.D. Lee and S.N. Blair, "Cardiorespiratory Fitness and Smoking-Related and Total Cancer Mortality in Men." *Medicine and Science in Sports and Exercise* 34(5) (May 2002): 735–39.

18. X. Sui, M.J. LaMonte, and S.N. Blair, "Cardiorespiratory Fitness as a Predictor of Nonfatal Cardiovascular Events in Asymptomatic Women and Men." *American Journal of Epidemiology* 165(12) (June 15, 2007): 1413–23.

19. P.N. Peterson, et al., "Association of Exercise Capacity on Treadmill with Future Cardiac Events in Patients Referred for Exercise Testing." *Archives of Internal Medicine* 168(2) (January 28, 2008): 174–79.

20. G.H. Guyatt, et al., "The 6-minute Walk: A New Measure of Exercise Capacity in Patients with Chronic Heart Failure." *Journal of the Canadian Medical Association* 132(8) (April 15, 1985): 919–23.

21. A.B. Newman, et al., "Association of Long-Distance Corridor Walk Performance with Mortality, Cardiovascular Disease, Mobility Limitation, and Disability." *Journal of the American Medical Association* 295(17) (May 3, 2006): 2018–26.

22. C. Bouchard, "Physical Inactivity." *Canadian Journal of Cardiology* 15(Supplement G) (December 1999): 89G–92G.

23. T.K. Fenske, M. Paletta, and B. Daub, "Exercising Your Post-MI Patient." *Patient Care* 12(9) (2001): 85–104.

24. M.B. Katan and N.M. de Roos, "Public Health: Toward Evidence-Based Health Claims for Foods." *Science* 299(5604) (January 10, 2003): 206–07.

25. A. Ascherio, "Trans Fatty Acids and Blood Lipids." *Atheroscler. Supplements* 7(2) (May 2006): 25–27. Epub May 19, 2006.

26. G.F. Watts, P.H. Barrett, and D.C. Chan, "HDL Metabolism in Context: Looking on the Bright Side." *Current Opinion in*

Lipidology 19(4) (August 2008): 395–404.

27. M. de Lorgeril, et al., "Mediterranean Diet, Traditional Risk Factors, and the Rate of Cardiovascular Complications after Myocardial Infarction: Final Report of the Lyon Diet Heart Study." *Circulation* 99(6) (February 16, 1999): 779–85.

28. T.K. Fenske, "Lipid-Lowering Update 2001. Aggressive New Goals." *Canadian Family Physician* 47 (February 2001): 303–09.

29. R. McPherson, et al. Canadian Cardiovascular Society. "Canadian Cardiovascular Society Position Statement — Recommendations for the Diagnosis and Treatment of Dyslipidemia and Prevention of Cardiovascular Disease." *Canadian Journal of Cardiology* 22(11) (September 2006): 913–27.

Chapter 8: Subtracting Addiction

1. J. Ambrose and R.S. Barua, "The Pathophysiology of Cigarette Smoking and Cardiovascular Disease: An Update." *Journal of the American College of Cardiology* 43 (2004): 1731–37.

2. H.K. Koh, L.X. Joosens, and G.N. Connolly, "Making Smoking History Worldwide." *New England Journal of Medicine* 356(15) (April 2007): 1496–98.

3. J. Cami and M. Farre, "Drug Addiction." *New England Journal of Medicine* 349(10) (September 2003): 975–86.

4. B. Le Foll and T.P. George, "Treatment of Tobacco Dependence: Integrating Recent Progress into Practice." *Journal of the Canadian Medical Association* 177(11) (2007): 1373–80.

5. K.A. Perkins, et al., "Metabolic Effects of Nicotine After Consumption of a Meal in Smokers and Nonsmokers." *American Journal of Clinical Nutrition* 52(2) (August 1990): 228–33.

6. S.A. Kenfield, et al., "Smoking and Smoking Cessation in Relation to Mortality in Women." *Journal of the American Medical Association* 299(17) (May 7, 2008): 2037–47.

7. T.F. Heatherton, et al., "The Fagerstrom Test for Nicotine Dependence: A Revision of the Fagerstrom Tolerance Questionnaire." *British Journal of Addictions* 86 (1991): 1119–27.

8. L.A. Jason, et al., "The Relationship Between Youth Tobacco Control Enforcement and Crime Rates in a Midwestern County." *American Journal of Health Promotion* 14(4) (March–April 2000): 229–31, iii.

9. J. Zarocostas, "WHO Report Warns Deaths from Tobacco Could Rise Beyond Eight Million a Year by 2030." *British Medical Journal* 336(7639) (February 9, 2008): 299.

10. M. Daniel, et al., "Cigarette Smoking, Mental Health and Social Support: Data from a Northwestern First Nation." *Canadian Journal of Public Health* 95(1) (January–February 2004): 45–49.

11. A.A. Wright and I.T. Katz, "Tobacco Tightrope — Balancing Disease Prevention and Economic Development in China." *New England Journal of Medicine* 356(15) (April 2007): 1493–96.

12. N.A. Rigotti, "Treatment of Tobacco Dependence." *New England Journal of Medicine* 346(7) (1997): 506–12.

13. J.T. Hays, "Tobacco Dependence Treatment in Patients with Heart and Lung Disease: Implications for Intervention and Re-

view of Pharmacological Therapy." *Journal of Cardiopulmonary Rehabilitation* 20 (2000): 215–23.

14. D.W. Wetter, et al., "Tobacco Withdrawal and Nicotine Replacement Influence Objective Measures of Sleep." *Journal of Consulting and Clinical Psychology* 63(4) (August 1995): 658–67.

15. S. Lam and P.N. Patel, "Varenicline: A Selective Alpha4beta2 Nicotinic Acetylcholine Receptor Partial Agonist Approved for Smoking Cessation." *Cardiology in Review* 15(3) (May–June 2007): 154–61. Review.

16. R.D. Hurt, et al., "A Comparison of Sustained-Release Buproprion and Placebo for Smoking Cessation." *New England Journal of Medicine* 337 (1997): 1195–1202.

17. S. Wilkes, "The Use of Bupropion SR in Cigarette Smoking Cessation." *International Journal of Chronic Obstructive Pulmonary Disorder* 3(1) (2008): 45–53. Review.

SELECTED
RESOURCES

Books

Carr, Allen. *The Easy Way to Stop Smoking*. New York: Sterling, 2005.

Vagnini, Frederic J., and Selene Yeager. *30 Minutes a Day to a Healthy Heart: One Simple Plan to Conquer All Six Major Threats to Your Heart*. New York: Reader's Digest, 2005.

Websites

Alternative Medicine
www.familydoctor.org
www.quackwatch.com

Blood Pressure

Canadian Hypertension Society (www.hypertension.ca)
www.heartandstroke.ca/bp

Diabetes

www.diabetes.ca

Diet

Canada's Food Guide (www.hc-sc.gc.ca) Food and Nutrition
(www.dieticians.ca)
DASH Diet (www.nih.gov)

Exercise

www.fitday.com
Health Canada physical activity guides (www.phac-aspc.gc.ca/
pau-uap/fitness/downloads.html)
www.healthtoolsonline.com/health-fit.html

Heart Health

www.capitalhealth.ca/EspeciallyFor/HeartSchool
www.cardiosmart.org
www.heartandstroke.ca
www.hearthub.org
www.nhlbi.nih.gov/health/public/heart
www.uptodate.com/patients

Mercury Consumption

www.ec.gc.ca (MERCURY/EN/fc.cfm)

Weight Loss

www.capitalhealth.ca/EspeciallyFor/WeightWise
www.obesitynetwork.ca
www.yourhealthyweight.ca

INDEX